Tatiana Ivanova

Depression in childhood

AF387211

Tatiana Ivanova

Depression in childhood

Ontogenesis and clinical dynamics

ScienciaScripts

Imprint

Any brand names and product names mentioned in this book are subject to trademark, brand or patent protection and are trademarks or registered trademarks of their respective holders. The use of brand names, product names, common names, trade names, product descriptions etc. even without a particular marking in this work is in no way to be construed to mean that such names may be regarded as unrestricted in respect of trademark and brand protection legislation and could thus be used by anyone.

Cover image: www.ingimage.com

This book is a translation from the original published under ISBN 978-3-8433-1320-9.

Publisher:
Sciencia Scripts
is a trademark of
Dodo Books Indian Ocean Ltd., member of the OmniScriptum S.R.L Publishing group
str. A.Russo 15, of. 61, Chisinau-2068, Republic of Moldova Europe
Printed at: see last page
ISBN: 978-620-3-06653-1

Copyright © Tatiana Ivanova
Copyright © 2021 Dodo Books Indian Ocean Ltd., member of the OmniScriptum S.R.L Publishing group

Table of contents

INTRODUCTION.

The problem of affective disorders in childhood and adolescence is one of the most actual in modern psychiatry in connection with frequency and "rejuvenation" of depressive disorders (I. V. Oleichik, 1998; L. V. Kim, 2006; N. M. Iovchuk, A. A. Severny, 2007; A. O. Adewuya, 2006). The depressive disorder which has begun in childhood is not only a predictor of high suicide risk (Slap G., Goodman E., 2001; Goldstein T. R, 2005), but also increases the possibility of depression (Pine D., Cohen P., Gurley D. et al., 1998; Biederman J., 2006) and other psychiatric disorders in adulthood (McCauley E. et al., 1993; Strober M. et al., 1993; Weissman M. et al., 2006). Significant growth of affective disorders in adults (Semke V.Y., Schastny E.D., Simutkin G.G., 2004) actualizes questions of studying depression in children. According to Russian and foreign researchers, the prevalence of depression by adolescence reaches 30%, and the average age of its occurrence is close to 9 years (Shevchenko Y. S., Iovchuk N. M., 1998; Kovacs M., Gatsonis C., 1994; Ivarsson T., 2006). It is necessary to note that the description of the clinical picture, nosological belonging and treatment approaches concern mainly depressive disorders of adolescence (Usov M. G., 1996; Antropov Y. F., 2001; Bohan N. A., Butorina N. E., Krivulin E. N., 2006; Weller E B., Kloos A., 2006).

The frequency of depressive states in the pediatric population in comparison to other psychopathological disorders varies widely, from 0.4-0.7% to 25% (Bomba J. et al., 1987; Hales D. P., Dishman R. K. et al., 2006; Blanchard L. T., 2006). However, it has been pointed out (Nissen G., 1987, et al.) that affective disorders in childhood occur much more frequently than they are diagnosed. Given the widespread occurrence of this pathology, the difficulties of qualifying, treating and rehabilitating these patients, and the serious medical and social prognosis, studying these issues is a highly relevant topic for practical healthcare. Difficulties of diagnostics of depressive disorders at the age of 6-14 years are connected with the fact that mental and physical development of the child's personality undergoes pronounced changes; this development is characterized by an original disharmony and unevenness, disturbance of the physiological and psychological balance achieved at the previous stage of ontogenesis (Shevchenko Y. S., Venger A. L., 2006; Gurieva V. A. et al., 2007).

Until now, depressive disorders in children have been studied within the framework of a particular nosological form: endogenous depression (V. Bashina. M., 1981; Mamtseva V. N., 1988; Golubeva N. I., Kozlovskaya G. F. 2001), organic depression (Isaev D. N., 1993; Gillberg K., Hellgren L., 2004), and depression in children with mental retardation (Gurieva V. A., 1996; Samarina E. V., 2007; Bortnick-Duffy S. A., 1990). The clinical typology of these disorders has not been developed up to this day and the connection between the psychopathological structure of the depressive syndrome and nosological identity has not been established. The questions of the "pathological basis" or dysontogenesis in children with the depressive syndrome (V.A. Gurieva, 2001) are practically not studied. In case studies (V. A. Gurieva, V. Y. Semke, V. Y. Gindikin, 1994) and in the works of psychologists (V. V. Lebedinsky, 1985) there is a point of view according to which understanding of age patterns of mental disorders and their diagnostics in children and teenagers is impossible without clear representation about correlations of clinic and disorders of mental development - dysontogenesis.

The present study was performed in the State Institution Research Institute of Mental Health, Tomsk Scientific Center of the Siberian Branch of the Russian Academy of Medical Sciences, State Educational Institution of Public Health "Clinical Psychiatric Hospital named after N.N. Solodnikov". N.N. Solodnikov Clinical Psychiatric Hospital. The clinical base of the study was the child-adolescent complex of the N.N. Solodnikov Omsk Clinical Psychiatric Hospital. N.N. Solodnikov. For realization of the purpose and tasks of the research we carried out clinical and follow-up and experimental-psychological examination of patients residing in Omsk and Omsk region who were treated in children departments of the mentioned medical preventive institution for depressive mood disorders during 5 years. The depressive symptoms were diagnosed in accordance with the clinical systematics DSM-IV and ICD-10, which was introduced into medical practice in 1993 according to the WHO decision. To identify children and adolescents with depressive disorders, most US researchers use the contemporary descriptions of depressive disorders presented in either the Diagnostic Criteria System manual (Spitzer R. L., Endicott J., Robins E., 1978) or the DSM-IV. Thus, the initial diagnosis of a depressive disorder in a child was made according to DSM-IV criteria, with subsequent qualification according to ICD-10.

Depressive disorders were considered in the following ICD-10 nosological categories: schizophrenia and schizoaffective disorders (F20-25); depressive behavioral disorders (F92); adjustment disorders, reactive depression (F43); mental retardation (F70-71).

Clinical-psychological testing was conducted using valid scales that had proven to be effective. According to the goals and objectives of the study, an original research protocol including three main directions was developed. Two validated scales recommended in pediatric practice were used to confirm the clinical diagnosis of depressive syndrome and to obtain a quantitative assessment of the severity of the mental state: the Child Depression Inventory - CDI (Kovacs M., Beck A. T., 1977) and the 21-item Hamilton Hospital Depression Scale.

Assessment of influence of the revealed depressive syndrome on socialization of the child was carried out with use of the Doll Scale of Social Competence (Doll E. A., 1953) as modified by V. I. Gordeev, Yu. S. Aleksandrovsky (2001), the essence of which is to simplify the procedure for calculation of the received result. Using this scale makes it possible to estimate the social age of the examinee (SA - social age), and on the basis of this the social quotient (SQ - social quotient) of the correlation between the social age and the chronological age. Each paragraph of the scale is labeled with age and category, which are subscales. SHG (selfhelpgeneral) - general self-care; SHE (selfhelp eating) - self-care in eating; SHD (selfhelp dressing) - self-care in dressing; SD (self-direction) - independence; O (occupation) - employment; C (communication) - communication; L (locomotion) - meaningful, purposeful movement; S (socialization) - socialization. Paragraphs of the scale are ranked in order of average age norms and are listed in an arithmetic series from 1 to 117, the ordinal number being the score to which a particular age corresponds. The protocol was filled out by the closest relatives (parents, grandparents), guardians, tutors.

The study sample of 341 patients with a verified diagnosis of depressive disorder was derived from the total population of patients undergoing inpatient treatment in the pediatric departments of the UCPB (3441 children) who had consulted a psychiatrist within 5 years. The spectrum of psychiatric pathology of the examined children was defined as "Organic emotionally labile disorder" (F06.6), "Organic personality disorder"   (F07.0),

"Mental   retardation"

(F70) and

"Behavioral, emotional, and conduct disorders beginning usually in childhood and adolescence" (F98).

Most psychiatrists believe that depressive disorders are a frequent component of many mental illnesses, influencing their essence and structure, with early identification of the nosological identity of the disorder necessary to determine prognosis and therapeutic approaches (Vrono M. Sh., 1979; Kovalev V. V., 1979; Vertogradova O. P., 1980, 1998; Tiganov A. S., Vidmanova L. N., Platonova T.

P., A. A. Sukhonsky, 1986; N. M. Iovchuk, 1989; S. N. Mosolov. N., 1995; Panteleeva G. P., 1999; Nissen G., 1972). The authors who share this opinion, when studying depression in adulthood, adolescence, adolescence and childhood, use the most traditional classification of P. Kielholz (1972), which is based on the nosological principle. It distinguishes organic, symptomatic, schizophrenic,

cyclical,

neurotic and reactive depression.

In Russian psychiatry, approaches to the study of affective pathology in adults and children coincide. In adults and young men, depressive states are described within the framework of schizophrenia, including schizoaffective psychoses, manic-depressive psychosis, neurotic disorders, reactive states and also in the structure of psychopathic personality development (Snezhnevsky A. V., 1968; Tsutsulkovskaya M. J., Panteleeva G. P., 1986; Vladimirova T. V., 1986; Vertogradova O. P., Voloshin V. M., 1989; Tiganov, A. S., 1997; Smulevich, A. B., 1997; Panteleeva, G. P., 1999). The psychiatrists studying depressive conditions in childhood and adolescence allocate, as a rule, the same nosological categories (Vrono M. Sh., 1971; Mamtseva V. N., 1982; Iovchuk N. M., 1986; Danilova L. Yu. V, 1995; Bashina V. M., 1999; Kozlova I. A., 1999), and distinctive

The specific features of childhood and adulthood are the different proportion of these nosological groups and their clinical manifestations.

Depressive disorders of predominantly neurotic nature prevailed in the study sample, which were revealed in 119 children (34.9%). Nosological affiliation of depression was defined as "Depressive spectrum adaptive disorder" (F43), "Depressive behavioral disorder" (F92). Depressions of organic nature were revealed in 110 patients (32.3%). Nosological affiliation of the disorder was defined as "Organic emotionally labile disorder" (F06.6) and "Organic personality disorder" (F07.0). Depression on the background of mental retardation was determined in 48 children (14.1%).

Endogenous depressive disorder was diagnosed in 18.7% of patients (n=64): "Schizophrenia, childhood type" (F20.8), "Schizotypal disorder" (F21) and "Schizoaffective disorder" (F25).

CHAPTER I.
THE PROBLEM OF DEPRESSIVE DISORDERS IN CHILDHOOD IN CONTEMPORARY PSYCHIATRY

1.1 The Emergence of Scientific Views on Childhood Depressive Disorders

In the pre-scientific period, the formation of a system of knowledge about the soul took place, and the signs of mental disorders were described mythologically in the spirit of the primitive-mythological worldview. The first attempts to provide medical care for the mentally ill appeared in the 6th or 7th century B.C., when diseases began to be regarded as a natural phenomenon requiring some kind of natural measures. The ancient philosophers Sophocles, Euripides, Socrates, Plato, Herodotus and Phidias contributed greatly to the study of mental disorders at that time. It was they who laid the conceptual foundations of scientific materialism when they expressed the idea that the cause of both healthy and sick person's behavior - "*psycho*" is within the body, somewhere in the depths of its tissues, in the matter of which it is composed.

They also set the stage for the brain theory, which Hippocrates later advanced: the brain is the organ of human cognition and adaptation to the environment: "We must know that, on the one hand, pleasures, joys, laughter, games and, on the other hand, sorrow, sadness, discontent and grievances come from the brain... It makes us insane, delirious, and we are seized by anxiety and fear." Thus arose the notion that mental illness, like all other diseases, has its anatomical localization. The Hippocratic books do not provide a complete and complete account of psychiatry. In various places - in Internal Diseases, Diseases of Young Women, Treatise on Diets, Epidemic Diseases, On Sacred Disease, and especially in Aphorisms - individual observations, theories, and therapeutic advice are scattered.

First in Hippocrates we find initial items In psychiatric terminology: melancholia, mania, phrenitis, paranoia, epilepsy. Calm states, generally speaking, were treated as melancholy, restless states as mania. Melancholics "are afraid of light and avoid people, they are full of all kinds of fears, complaining of stomach pains, as if they were pricked by thousands of tiny needles. Sometimes they have difficult dreams, and in reality they see images of the dead. But melancholy in Hippocrates has not one but two meanings: it is, firstly, the disease that manifests itself just listed symptoms, and secondly, it is a special temperament, a special constitution with a humoral basis and psychological characteristics. Melancholic temperament is characterized by a predominance of timidity, reticence, sadness. On the basis of this temperament is often the disease itself: "If feelings of fear or cowardice last too long, it points to the onset of melancholy. "Fear and sadness, if they last a long time and are not caused by worldly reasons, come from black bile.

This was the first stage in the development of child psychiatry, which Kannibach (1929) would later call "negative", since the possibility of mental disorder in a child was simply denied. This negative attitude was fundamental. Psychosis was believed to be the sad privilege of a person who had already experienced the difficulties of life and the fatal influence of passions (Kraus, 1809). Even from a functional point of view, it was argued that the elementary and comparative simplicity of brain acts guaranteed children against mental illness. Idiocy and cretinism were deliberately ignored as congenital conditions of little social or therapeutic interest. The violent states sometimes observed in defective children were seen as a complication of their underlying disorder. Among mental disorders in children, only conditions comparable to modern oligophrenia are distinguished.

Felix Plater (1589) described "congenital insanity, or stupidity - "*siuliilia*" of children from the first years of life, representing various signs of defectiveness: they are disobedient, obstinate, hard to learn to speak, lacking intelligence in the simplest things; in addition, they are marked by physical defects: the wrong shape of the head, the manner of eating, the specificity of their gestures, speech defects". In the VII-VIII centuries, works concerning the basic principles of defectology and psychopathology of childhood appear. In particular, Segen (1852) has described a way to improve elementary functions of sensory and motor apparatuses of defective children (vision, hearing, quickness and dexterity, motor functions); education, in his opinion, should be as concrete as possible, and represent a "school of things". Segen's thoughts (1852) are set forth in his monograph: "Upbringing, Hygiene and Moral Treatment of Mentally Defective Children.

However, from the beginning of the 19th century, some casuistic observations that were at variance with this categorical view began to be published. It began to be admitted that fear, acute pains, strong overexertion, head bruises can, though in rather rare cases, lead to real psychoses in children. In 1825. Kasper in his book "Medical Statistics" already gives figures of suicides of children; the latter are considered by him as the result of the strongest griefs caused by offenses, punishments, etc.; at the same time ideas about the possibility of melancholy in childhood are already beginning to form. Zeller (1846) suggested that children have quite the same course of mental illness as adults, namely, that the initial melancholy turns into mania and then into dementia. In later years a significant step forward was the work of J. Moreau de Tours (1888): "Hallucination in childhood. This ended the second stage of the history of child psychiatry, which can be called a period of scattered instructions and unsystematized casuistry.

The third stage begins with the work of the English pediatrician Z. West (Emmingnaus G., 1887). He describes in children besides dementia and epilepsy also "true lunacy", besides various mood abnormalities, quite the same as in adults, but only proceeding in milder forms. At the same time the number of casuistic reports of psychoses in childhood increases rapidly. And in 1864 a monograph by Berkan was published. This author collected 55 cases of psychoses in children under 12 years of age, categorized under the following headings:

melancholia, mania, hallucinatory insanity, and dementia. Berkan's work (1864) completes the third stage; now psychoses in childhood become an incontrovertible and proven fact.

The fourth stage marked its beginning with the publication of H. Maudsley's (1871) monograph Physiology and Pathology of the Soul. This work, according to H. Emminghaus (1887), serves as a turning point in the history of child psychiatry. H. Maudsley (1871) pointed to age as an etiological moment, systematized and formalized everything known before him, and proposed the following classification of child psychoses: 1) monomania (murder, suicide, arson, theft), 2) delirium in chorea, with peculiar confusion, frequent hallucinations, and various kinds of automatic symptoms, 3) cataleptic lunacy, 4) epileptic lunacy, 5) mania, 6) melancholia 7) affective, or moral lunacy.

The modern era in the history of child psychiatry begins with a major scientific achievement, the book by N. Emminghaus, The Mental Disorders of Childhood. (1887). The author distinguishes the following diseases in children: 1) cerebral neurasthenia, 2) melancholia with suicidal tendencies, 3) mania, 4) acute dementia, 5) hypochondria, 6) paranoia, 7) obsessive thoughts, 8) transient insanity, 9) periodic insanity, 10) moral insanity, 11) idiocy, 12) epilepsy. In parallel with the theoretical advances of this new direction in psychiatry, children's departments in hospitals rapidly spread and improved. Independent institutions were opened in Moscow: a treatment school for mentally ill children, founded by O. B. Feltsman (1915), and the model clinic of the Second Moscow State University, established under the direction of Professor V. A. Gilyarovsky (1922).

The study of depression in children emerged at the turn of the 19th-20th centuries. Thus, in the first half of the 19th century, works on "casuistic" cases of melancholy in children were first published, but the scientific descriptions at that time were of an individual clinical publication (Pinel Ph., 1809). However, with the development of child psychiatry and the opening of specialized pediatric departments, the study of childhood depression began to gradually acquire a systematic character. After the opening of the specialized children's department in Bictre (1850-1860), the number of observations of mentally ill children increased, the first attempts to generalize clinical material appeared. Delasiauve (1840, 1864) was the first to describe the main features of depressive conditions in children and the principles of their treatment. Subsequently, in the widely popular monographs of W. Griesinger (1886), H. Maudsley (1871), H. Emminghaus (1887), J. Moreau de Tours (1888), E. Kraepelin (1913), T. Ziehen (1917) provided vivid clinical descriptions of childhood melancholy, hypochondria, anxiety-excited depression.

In particular, W. Griesinger (1868) pointed out that children and adolescents, although quite rare, still have melancholic states, but they are based on a feeling of general restlessness and anxiety. And children's suicides, in his opinion, are a consequence of a distorted, differently proceeding melancholy than in adults. Zeller, West (1887) believed that children, as well as adults, might have mood abnormalities. In 1867 Maudsley, in his book devoted entirely to child psychiatry, for the first time provided a classification of mental illnesses in children, including such independent nosological units as melancholia and mania.

In 1887 H. Emminqhaus distinguished in children simple melancholy, melancholy with anxiety, melancholy with frantic perceptions, and melancholy with torpor. A sad mood, in his opinion, is always a symptom of illness if it occurs without mental reason and lasts for a long time. As the basic symptoms of melancholy of childhood the author named such as seclusion, brooding, detachment, tearfulness, "confusion", agitation up to raptus melancholicus, ideas of self-blame. H. Emminqhaus (1890) emphasized that in children with melancholy, the initiative is strong only in relation to their complaints, self-blame and self-abasement. He also noted an increased tendency "to illness, fears, fright and other depressing feelings" (1890, p. 67). According to the degree of severity, the author distinguished three degrees of "voluntary melancholy" in children occurring for no definite reason: mild, severe and the highest. In describing this symptomatology, he drew attention to the rarity of localization of melancholy in the pre-cardiac area and the absence in children of "wandering inner melancholy" and "melancholy arising from the forehead" (*Dysthymia frontalis, lyriesinqer*). In the majority of observations, melancholia was accompanied by sleep disorders, appetite, constipation, tachycardia and, in severe cases, pronounced symptoms of intoxication. All the main manifestations of the disease appeared in the morning, and in rare cases, deterioration occurred in the afternoon. The author described as a characteristic feature of melancholy in children "the alternation of remissions and exasperations" (p. 64), which disappeared with prolonged melancholy, and of increasing mental sadness. In addition to prolonged (from several months to several years) melancholy in a child, the author also distinguished in some cases acute, lightning-fast melancholy.

Moreau de Tours (1888) subdivided "mental depression" into hypochondria, delirium of persecution, melancholia, and stupor as a type of melancholia. The main difference between depressive states in children and similar states in adults, according to the author, is the naive subject matter and indistinctness of depressive, hypochondriac delirium and delirium of persecution; in the basic manifestations they do not differ from depression in adults.

The Homburger (1926) manual and the Strohmaeyer (1926) lectures, in addition to brilliant descriptions of the phenomenology of childhood melancholy and mania, already contained clear nosological and differential diagnostic criteria, supplemented by recommendations for the treatment and management of pediatric patients. Hombyrger (1926) considered fear, tendency to stupor, complaints of pain and discomfort in various parts of the body, crying replacing complaints of longing, "miserable expression" of feelings, laziness, and poor academic performance to be typical features of depressive states in children. He also noted not only the frequency of self-blaming ideas, but also accusations and reproaches directed at others, lies, unkindness toward brothers and sisters. According to the author's observations, the duration of depressions in children ranged from several days to several months, and their main distinguishing feature was their rapid onset and slow recovery.

Russian psychiatrists at the beginning of the 20th century also studied features of the depressive syndrome in childhood. V. A. Gilyarovsky (1935), A. I. Vinokurova (1935) and S. S. Mukhin (1940) thought that manic-depressive psychosis in childhood was much more common than is commonly thought, but was not diagnosed, since the phases were poorly expressed, dull, indistinct and were diagnosed as "simple nervousness". A. I. Vinokurova (1935) thought that depression in childhood was even relatively more common than in puberty and the early period thereafter.

Fear, anxiety and tendency to obsessions dominate in the clinic of childhood depression. In almost all children with depression vegetative disorders are significantly expressed, often depression is accompanied by enuresis (V. A. Gilyarovsky, 1955; S. S. Mukhin, 1940).

Subsequently, interest in childhood affective disorders declined somewhat and resumed only since the second half of the 20th century, when new research works in this area appeared. In part, this interest was provoked by an increase in depressive disorders among children due to the social disadvantages of those years (social and economic reforms, a large number of international wars and conflicts). Thus, since the middle of the 50's of the last century, interest in this problem again grows, there are works devoted already to the clinical formulation (Lapides M.I., 1940; Mayer-Gross W., Slater E., Roth M., 1954) and age features of the mostly depressive syndrome (Sukhareva G.E., 1955; Krevclen D.A., 1972).

M. I. Lapides (1940), in describing circular depression in children, draws attention to a different type of daily fluctuations than in adult patients, a worsening of mood in the evening and the presence in the clinical picture of somatic manifestations - headaches, general weakness, a tendency to constipation and loss of body weight. W. Mayer-Gross, E. Slater, M. Roth (1954) emphasize the rarity of depressive states in the childhood period. However, the authors point out that fearfulness, dysmnesic complaints, concentration difficulties in schoolchildren can still be evidence of depressive reactions, so well known in adult patients, and believe that the main role in the origin of such depressions is played by psychogenic factors.

In spite of the fact that R. A. Spitz in 1946 described the manifestations of depression in young children, up to the 70s of the 20th century the problem of childhood and adolescent depression was not paid much attention in the foreign thematic literature. This is explained by a number of factors, the most significant of which is considered to be the dominance of the psychoanalytic view of depression as a condition that cannot occur in an individual without the presence of a mature superego.

In the 1960s, the understanding of the nature and treatment of depression in adults was predominantly viewed from the standpoint of the biologization approach in psychiatry (Ballenger J. C., 1988), in the 1970s a number of cognitive and behavioral models of depression (Craighead W. E., 1980) are already emerging.

The development of the theory of depression, both empirically and conceptually, as opposed to the psychoanalytic viewpoint, allowed the possibility of depression in childhood and adolescence, which led to an extraordinary interest in its study. An analysis of the research of that period by G. A. Carlson (1980), allows considering that all symptoms of depression exhibited in adults, can often be observed in adolescents and even in children.

Since the mid-1970s, there have been papers showing that affective disorders occur much more frequently than they are diagnosed (Spiel W., 1972; Puig-Antich J., Goetz D. et al., 1989).

As early as 1970, the French psychiatrist J. D. Ajuriaguerra published his first manual on child psychiatry, which covers the problem of affective disorders in children in a rather comprehensive way. In the work the peculiarities of child depression are described: "...up to pubertal age one can find in some children a particular symptomatology characterized by a state of sadness, indifference, melancholy and despair, a feeling of worthlessness with ideas of physical disappearance, a picture similar to the one classically defined as depression in adults". However the author does not insist on "inevitable inclusion" of such variant of depression into the category of classical melancholy (Ajuriaguerra J. D., 1970).

There was no unanimity in questions concerning the age of manifestation of depressive disorders. Some researchers (Ushakov G.K., 1973; Kovalev V.V., 1995) considered depressive disorders only within the framework of manic-depressive psychosis and claimed that the occurrence of endogenous depression is impossible earlier than 12 years. Nevertheless, the results of epidemiological studies by M. Kovacs, C. Catsonis (1994) showed that in children born in 1969-1970, the mean age of the first episode of major depressive disorder was 11.6 years, and in those born in 1975 - 9.9 years. These results confirmed the well-known position of Kraepelin, who as early as 1904 believed that it was possible to recognize endogenous depression before the age of 10. His opinion in subsequent years was shared by many psychiatrists (Campbell J. D., 1952; Anthony Y., Scott P., 1960; Kuhn R., 1963; Spiel W., 1964; Wieck Ch., 1965; Stutte H., 1972). Moreover, T. P. Simpson (1958), A. N. Chekhova (1968), V. V. Kovalev (1995), G. Nissen (1975), V. M. Bashina (1989) describe rather typical displays of depressive symptomatology in children, starting from an early age. The majority of researchers engaged in depressions, first of all, have specified considerable frequency of their manifestation at pubertal age (Sukhareva, G. E., 1955; Vertogradova O. P., 1980; Lichko A. E., 1985; Northern A. A., 1985; Stutte H., 1972).

At present in the foreign thematic literature there are a number of points of view on childhood and adolescent depression, including such a view as its complete denial. There are five directions in the study of childhood depressive disorders (Carlson G. A., Garber J., 1986), two of which have been considered the most significant in the past. The first is based on psychoanalytic theories of personality development and denies the existence of a full-fledged clinical syndrome of mood disorders due to underdevelopment of the super-ego in adolescents.

In the 1960s and 1970s, this view established the theory of masked depression, according to which manifestations such as delinquent behaviors, somatic complaints or lack of parental control could be symptoms of a specified dynamically motivated depressive state. The advantages of this theory include, first, that it emphasizes the need for professionals to be more attentive to affective disorders in children and adolescents that do not fit into the mood disorders and thus fall out of control, and second, that it has paved the way for more specific models of depression in adolescents.

One objection to the theory of masked depression is that, in fact, most psychological phenomena in children can be considered within the framework of generation or reflection of depressive states, and thus none of the groups of disorders appears out of connection with the state of depression (Kovacs M., Beck A. T., 1977). On a more pragmatic level, careful research on depressive symptoms has shown that many types of masked behaviors are fairly "transparent masks" and that the presence of a depressive syndrome can be ascertained directly through interviews (Carlson G. A., Cantwell D. P., 1980).

This has led to the modern view that depression is often accompanied by other disorders, but these are more often defined as comorbid conditions rather than as depressive sequelae or protective masks. More recent schools representing the second school understand childhood and adolescent depression as a clinical form of disorder, but do not agree with the clinical treatment of its essential features (Carlson G. A., Garber J., 1986). The scientific activity of the third school is associated with the names of scientists W. A. Weinberg (1973) and his colleagues (Weiberg W. A., Rutman J., Suillivan L. et al., 1973), who described the depressive syndrome in children as a combination of several symptoms identical to those of depression in adults, combined with specific symptoms that characterized the child during ontogenesis. Nevertheless, the most influential and authoritative, underlying most modern currents is the fourth school, which recognizes essential similarity of childhood and adult depressive disorders, despite some clinical and dynamic features (Puig- Antich J., Weston B., 1983). This position has led researchers to use a conventional set of criteria, of the DSM-

III type, when defining depressive disorders over an individual's lifetime.

Despite the fact that this approach has led to greater productivity in research of early depressive disorders, it has been criticized by representatives of the fifth school mainly for the fact that it did not take into account the influence of features of child development, their capabilities and limitations in manifestation of symptomatology (Cicchetti D., Schneider-Rosen K, 1986). According to this fifth view, often identified with developmental psychopathology, age-specific features of depressive symptomatology were examined and significant features of its developmental manifestation were identified.

Now presence of depressive disorders in children is proved (Mamtseva V. N., 1982; Iovchuk N. M., Severny A. A., 1999; Alderman J., Wolkov R., Chung M. et. al., 1998; Adewuya A. O., 2006), however descriptions of the clinical picture, nosological belonging and approaches to treatment concern mainly depressions occurring in teenagers, that is probably connected with more typical clinical picture and high prevalence of the specified mood disorders in teenagers (Dmitrieva T. B., 1981; Gurieva V. A., Gindikin V. Ya. Y., V. Y. Semke, 1994; I. V. Oleichik, 1998; Y. F. Antropov, 2001).

1.2. Prevalence of depression among children

The possibility of occurrence in childhood of dysthymic states comparable with affective syndromes of adults was not recognized by all psychiatrists (Rumke H. C., 1928; Corboz R., 1958; Rie H. E., 1966; Asperger H., 1969); many psychiatrists considered them extremely rare, others insisted on a high incidence of these disorders, although they recognized their "masked" character. According to these views, the frequency of depressive states in comparison to other psychopathological disorders varies in a wide range from 0.4-0.7 to 25% in the child population. However, many authors (Kuhn R., 1963; Spiel W., 1969; Ajuriaguerra J., 1970; Mcirhofer M., 1972; Nissen G., 1987) emphasize that affective disorders in childhood occur much more frequently than are diagnosed.

The prevalence of depression among mental disorders of childhood and in the general population, according to various authors, varies enormously. Thus, J. Witkowska-Roszka (1980) defined depression in 2 % of patients of the child psychiatric hospital, R. Kuhn (1963) - in 12,4 %, M. Negri, G. Moretti (1972), D. A. Waller, J. A. Rush (1983) - in 19%, even higher figures are given by D. P. Cantwell (1983) and S. G. Hershberg et al. (1982) - in 27 %, R. W. Gibson (1978) - in 33 %.

G. Nissen (1973) diagnosed depression in 11% of stateless children and adolescents between the ages of 6 and 20. In his opinion, the most frequent (50%) depressive disorders occur at the age of 11-14 years, while at the primary school age the number of depressions is 2 times less, and at the infant and preschool age depressions are extremely rare at all. According to the data cited by J. B. Weiner (1970) and J. H. Kashani et al. (1982), depression is significantly more common among general inpatients (12-16%) than among outpatients and psychiatric inpatients (3.8% and 3.7%, respectively).

In a population study, depression in childhood was detected by W. Schmitz (1979) in 0.03% of cases, A. Weber (1955) in 3%, M. Mcierhofer (1972) in 25%, N. Albert and A. T. Beck (1975) in 33.3%. J. Bomba et al. (1987) in their study of a population of children and adolescents found that depression was present in 6.66% of observations in 5-year-olds, in 11.3% in 10-year-olds, and was sharply more frequent by puberty (in 31.6% of children in early puberty). According to D. R. Robbins et al. (1988), the prevalence of adolescent depression in the clinical population ranges from 5 to 33%.

One of the most wide-ranging studies of childhood depression was conducted by C. Z. Garrison et al. (1992). The CESDS (Center for Epidemiologic Studies Depression Scale) questionnaire was used as a screening method among 3283 schoolchildren in the United States 12-14 years old, and the Schedule for Affective Disorders and Schizophrenia in School Age Children, based on DSM-III diagnostic criteria, was used as a clinical interview at the second stage. The prevalence of severe depressive disorder was found to be 9.04% for boys and

8.90% for girls, and of dysthymia, 7.98% and 5%, respectively.

In a large, comprehensive, single-stage, questionnaire-based study in Canada in 1983 (The Ontario Childe Health Study), the prevalence of severe depressive disorder among pre-pubertal children ranged from 1.8% to 7.8%, and 43%, depending on the degree of compliance with the diagnostic test. (The Ontario Childe Health Study), the prevalence of major depressive disorder among pre-pubertal and pubertal children ranged from 1.8% to 7.8% and 43.9%, depending on the degree to which the DSM-III diagnostic criteria were met. In a 2-stage population-based study of 11- to 16-year-old girls (n=1072), the prevalence of clinical level depressive disorder was 8.9%, with 3.6% of cases identifying moderate to severe depression (DSM-III). In the 2003 Child Mental Health Assessment conducted by American psychiatrists, depressive disorders in children 6-17 years old were found in 36% of those surveyed (Blanchard L. T., 2003). Diagnostic errors associated with depression are based, according to R. Kuhn (1963) and G. Nissen (1973) that the syndromal qualification criteria for depression in adults cannot be transferred to a child because the phenomenology of childhood depression is defined by the "time factor" (Erammer W., 1964), which plays a pathoplastic role in the typical preformation of depressive syndromes over a lifetime.

1.3. Causes of depression in childhood

In a paper of 1888, P. Moreau de Tours summarized the findings on childhood mental illnesses. In his opinion, "heredity is one of the most undiscussable predispositions, which is found always, in all the cases we have registered. It constitutes the main cause, as necessary in the development of insanity as provocation by purely accidental causes" (p. 295). Among provoking causes the author lists as the most important traumatism, especially craniocerebral injuries, poisoning by poisonous substances, onanism, psychotraumatic moments, the beginning of menstruation, worm infestation (Moreau de Tours P., 1877, 1888).

In the aspect of psychoanalytical concepts the essence of depression is interpreted as the repression of "Ego" in connection with the conflict of "Ego" and conscience. According to J. Wiesse, P. Mattejat (1881-1882), M. Harrington, J. Hassan (1959), D. B. Rinsley (1965), because Ego function is not yet established in childhood, a full-fledged "dialogue of guilt and redemption" is not possible, which provides an argument for claiming the extreme rarity of childhood depression. The emergence of depression in childhood can be explained as a result of the destruction of the "Ego" function with the loss of cognitive processes and corresponding processes of restitution, conflict because of insufficient contact with the mother at an early age (Statten T., 1961) or improper development of personality because of the long-term imbalance between the coexisting impulses of love and hatred.

Proponents of psychodynamic concepts (Bradley C., 1949; Cassullo A. G., Fabiani M. E., 1972; Tincoloni V. G., Toschi P., 1972; Lebovici S., 1972; Katz J., 1979) consider depression in the child from positions of natural mental development as a result of loss (real or existing in fantasies) of a beloved object, and the feeling of impossibility of existence without it. P. A. Murray (1970), J. Varsamis, S. M. McDonald (1972), I. Biermann, B. Pflug (1974) in describing children with distinct bipolar phases with obvious hereditary MDP burden, see the cause of the affective phases in lack of love in early childhood, although they note that in adulthood the transition of manic-depressive phases into MDP is possible. This interpretation is opposed by W. M. Rey (1980), who specifically studied 231 patients with MDD at an advanced age and has not established any correlations between decrease of parental love and age at the moment of manifestation of psychosis, argues against such an interpretation.

The psychodynamic theories are based on the teachings of M. Klein (1934, 1944, 1948), concerning, as well as the works of R. A. Spitz (1967), concerning infancy. Under the name "depressive stance" M. Klein described a "universal phenomenon" peculiar to the development of the normal child between 3 and 5 months of life. The mother in this phase is a source of both good and bad, as a result of which the child has a feeling of internal weakness and dependence, and the child's position in the relationship with the mother is ambivalent. During the depressive phase, according to M. Klein (1944), there is a fear of persecution and anxiety concentrated on the fear of own destructive actions, due to which the infant feels despair, grief for the lost object and self-blame for its destruction.

R. A. Spitz (1946) sharply opposed the theory of M. Klein (1944), believing that depression in an infant cannot be spoken of as a characteristic "psychosis of childhood development" and that depression in early childhood can only be a consequence of some frustrations.

A. I. Modina (1971) names the following among the reasons for negative emotions and formation of low moods in children: 1) disruption of the habitual stereotype of behavior (change of environment or social circle); 2) improper construction of the child's daily routine;   3) improper educational techniques; 4) lack of necessary conditions for play; 5) creation of one-sided affective attachment; 6) lack of a unified approach to the child.

Regarding psychogenic factors contributing to mood changes in children, J. Heisel et al. (1973) name more than 30 reasons leading to emotional distress and development of depression. Of them the most significant in preschool and younger school age are death, divorce, separation of parents, and in high school age - pregnancy.

In discussing the connection of depression in a child with external factors, R. Kuhn (973, p. 88) writes, "General psychiatric experience shows that healthy children are more robust than we tend to assume; therefore, unfavorable environmental conditions affect especially unhealthy children, whether cyclothymic disturbances, intellectual and characteristic abnormalities or organic brain damage are involved," thus arguing for the role of psychogenia in children as a trigger factor for depression.

Г. E. Sukhareva (1955, 1959) mentioned a great number of vegetosomatic disorders in the clinic of psychogenic depressions. Depression as a result of chronic psychological trauma (failure at school, loss of close people, separation from them) is characterized by low intensity of melancholy, the prevalence of phenomena of heightened sensitivity, vulnerability and emotional instability.

The author believes that in order to diagnose these depressive conditions, a number of specific features must be taken into consideration: 1) they occur against a background of a pronounced asthenic condition; 2) clinical manifestations are characterized by great lability; 3) in the clinical picture of illness there is a connection with a psychotraumatic situation.

An even less solved, but very urgent problem in child psychiatry is the possibility of the occurrence of depressive states in infancy. The cause of infant depression is mainly seen in the factors of "separation", "frustration" and "deprivation" (Lanhmeier J., Matejcek Z., 1984), existing in the separation from the mother or in her

Insolvency. Until now, the attention of child psychiatrists has been attracted by a particular syndrome in infants described by R. A. Spitz (1960) called "anaclitic depression" of long-term observation of children completely separated from their mothers and experiencing emotional deficit. After separation from the mother, children who until then had been active, cheerful, trusting, sociable, became tearful, fearful, irritable, stopped actively playing. The resistance stage gave way to the exhaustion stage: loss of interest in others progressed, tearfulness disappeared, autoerotic activity joined in. The infant's condition resembled a lethargic sleep, insomnia, a sharp decrease in appetite or refusal of food, weight loss, as well as an increase in the propensity to respiratory diseases and eczema were noted. Such conditions were observed by R. A. Spitz (1946) between 6 and 11 months of life and were reversible if the child was returned to the mother within 3 months. Otherwise there was an irreversible syndrome of infantile hospitalism with rough disturbance of psychomotor development and a picture of "stuporous catatonia" or "agitated idiocy".

According to studies of social risk factors in the occurrence of depression in children and adolescents, due to the identified correlations, different socio-demographic, psychological, and family indicators were given the status of potentially depressogenic. In particular, correlations with such factors as age, gender, ethnicity, socio-economic status, type of family dysfunction, stresses during life, presence of psychopathology in parents, low intellectual level, presence of somatic diseases, low self-esteem were studied (Adewuya A. O., 2006).

In a study by D. B. Kandel, M. Davies (1982) studied the relationship of depression to various socio-demographic, psychological characteristics on a sample of children. According to these researchers, the lowest probability of depression was found in children and adolescents whose relationships with parents were characterized as warm, trusting, and with peers as active. The higher the level of peer inclusion, the lower the likelihood of depression. Children and adolescents from authoritarian families and families where one parent was depressed had a much higher risk of depression. Other factors, such as race, religious beliefs, and social level, were not found to correlate with depression.

By now there is a lot of evidence that inadequate behavior of the mother during pregnancy, her emotional reactions to the stresses of her life cause a significant number of different pathological conditions in the child, both behavioral, psychological and somatic (Batuev A.S., Sokolova L.V., 1994; Batuev A.S., 2000). The mother's attitude towards the fetus during pregnancy leaves persistent traces on the development of its psyche (Fries M. E., 1987). Emotional stress correlates with premature birth, a large child psychopathology, more frequent occurrence of schizophrenia, often with school failures, high rates of delinquency, propensity for drug abuse and suicide attempts (R.J. Mukhamedrakhimov, 1994; Fereira A., 1980; L.R. Negren, 1982; Ward A.J., 1991). Trauma of a fetus can be reflected in the affective sphere of the adult (Edelton G., 1989).

1.4 Clinical and Dynamic Characteristics of Depressive Disorders in Children

Since E. Kraepelin (1904), a depressive state has been characterized by the so-called depressive triad: low mood, motor and mental retardation. Depressive triad with holistic and harmonious inhibition in all links is still given great importance as a diagnostic sign of endogenous depression (Vertogradova O. P. Voloshin V. M., 1989; Tiganov A. S., 1997; Panteleeva G. P., 1999). The basic links of the triad are well enough studied in the description of depression in adults, although certain disagreements concerning the basic components of the triad do not allow to consider this question definitively resolved (Nuller J. L., 1988; Smulevich A. B. et al., 1997, 1998; Tiganov A. S., 1999).

G. Nissen (1971, 1972) identified five different judgments about depression in childhood: 1) depressive disorders in childhood are not known; 2) every childhood depression is a masked depression; 3) depressive disorders in children are not different from depressive disorders in adults; 4) depressive disorders never occur under the label of depressive disorders in adults; 5) depressive disorders in children reveal specific psychosomatic and hypochondriacal symptoms. In order to clarify the symptomatology of depression in children and adolescents, G. Nissen (1971, 1972) conducted clinical and statistical research and identified the 5 most frequent psychiatric symptoms (insecure contacts, fear, stiffness, isolation, insecurity) and 5 psychosomatic symptoms (aggressiveness, bedwetting, sleep disturbance, mutism, nail nibbling).

On the basis of statistical calculations of occurrence of these or those signs, it was concluded that girls with a depressive disorder are as a rule whiny, quiet, constrained, inclined to mood swings, brooding, and boys are inclined to isolation and uncommunicative, irritability and difficulties in school behavior (Nissen G., 1971). The author has also noted characteristic distinctions in symptomatology of depressive conditions in various age groups - preschoolers show psychosomatic symptoms (fits of crying, crying, encopresis, sleep disorders, appetite) and teenagers show psychic and psychosomatic symptoms of adults, indicating mainly "intrapsychic conflicts. To the category of "intrapsychic conflicts" G. Nissen (1971) lists suicidal tendencies, inferiority complexes, depression and headaches. Of the diagnostic syndromes derived by paired symptom compounds, the most common was "stiffly" depressed (66%), with "agitatedly" depressed in second place (27%) and "mixed" in third place (8%). As diagnostically unfavorable symptoms, G. Nissen (1972) referred to delirium, dysphoria, suicide attempts, sadness, mutism.

According to M. de Negri, G. Moretti (1972), in case of depression in the "first childhood", somatic disorders (nutrition, sleep) and development disorders prevail. At preschool age, depression is manifested by mental retardation (sometimes to the point of pseudo-debility), lack of initiative, limited contact, tendency to isolation, bouts of crying, negative reactions to frustration, onset of autoeroticism, regressive states (enuresis), phobias or anxiety. At school age, depression is revealed by an increase in auto- and hetero-aggressiveness, stable autoerotic behavior, decreased school adaptation, phobias, anxiety. The authors made the following conclusions: 1) childhood depression is associated with environmental factors, i.e., it is always reactive; 2) endogenous pathogenesis can be found indirectly (pathological heredity, apparent lack of motivation); 3) prolonged anxiety can lead to paroxysmal phenomena (nightmares, seizures of suffocation, etc.), less often - to a persistent condition of emotional tension; 4) there is almost never a typical ideational depressive pathology (ideas of destruction, guilt); fantastic phobias are very close to physiological fears; 5) the childhood depression is easily changed under the influence of external environment; 6) the childhood suicides have sharp emotional pathogenesis (on the type of "short circuit").

To determine the characteristics of childhood and adolescent depression, G. Nissen (1982) conducted a clinical and statistical study of 105 depressed pediatric inpatients. Among age-specific clinical features, the author noted the following pattern. At preschool age, psychosomatic disorders are mostly detected, in junior high school - "mental symptoms with strong affective involvement" (excitable, shy, irritable, "quiet child"), in adolescence - "adult mental and psychosomatic disorders indicating predominantly intrapsychic conflicts" (lying, suicidal tendencies, inferiority complex, depression, headaches). Wistfulness, longing, mutism were singled out as prognostically unfavorable symptoms, and a single sign - "mood swings" - was pathognomic for further development of the schizophrenic process.

A. Weber (1973), studying the causes of depression in young children and in prepubertal children, assumes that they are different. In the first case, depression is a consequence of the broken intrafamilial relations in systems "mother-child" and "father-child". In the second case, depressive disorders are a result of school overload. The main clinical signs of childhood depression are apathy, indifference or some negativism, anorexia, tearfulness, and aspiration to be quiet and invisible.

Г. Е. Sukhareva (1955), revealing problems of children's affective pathology, notes, that in the clinical picture of depression the great specific weight belongs to vegetative-somatic disorders. Unpleasant somatic sensations, pain in the heart region, and in young children - abdominal pain are common complaints of such patients. The author emphasizes that these age-specific features of depressions nevertheless make one think first of the presence of a somatic, rather than mental illness in a child.

Г. К. Ushakov (1973) identifies the following symptoms of affective disorders typical for childhood: anaclitic depression (a state of extreme passivity, expressed apathy), night terror, emotional movement anxiety, nervous skin itching, emotional anorexia, childhood dysphoria. Common features of childhood affective symptoms, according to the author, are comparatively short-term, fleeting, erased states of depression; a greater mismatch than in adults, between the occasion and severity of emotional reactions; polymorphism of types of affective reactions; coexistence of rudiments of emotional disorders with motor, autonomic and obsessive reactions. It is marked, that since teenage years, especially since 13-14 years, in the clinical picture of mental illnesses, along with the listed symptoms of affective disorders, typical for adults, but in more erased, rudimentary form, more often occur. In the clinic of depression there is no feeling of despair, the feeling of longing weakens, elements of dysphoria or apathy with the phenomena of lethargy, sleep disorders, appetite prevail; tearfulness, motor stiffness, lethargy prevail.

There are different syndromological taxonomies of depressive disorders in children, which have no unified grouping criteria and separately do not reflect the variety of phenomenological variants of depression. Most commonly, depressive states were divided according to the predominant affect in the clinical picture. H. Kielholz, C. Adams (1980) divided depression into four main forms: with melancholy and depression, with anxiety and agitation, apathetic forms and larvic conditions with neurovegetative and psychosomatic symptoms. Some systematics have used both syndromological and nosological categories. For example, M. Schachter (1972) distinguished "melancholic states", "depressive preschizophrenic states", "neurotic" and "mixed states." C. Kohler, F. Bernard (1970, 1972) made an attempt to systematize previously described depressive states and distinguished "melancholic states", "depressive preschizophrenic states", "reactive depressive states", "mixed difficult to differentiate states", "depression caused by organic reasons and school overload".

There is a division of depression according to the preceding stressful event. In particular, J. M. Toolan (1971) divides childhood depression into anaclitic depression, depression in children of depressed mothers, depression in parental divorce, depression with intellectual disability, masked depression and anorexia with depression. M. Kovacs (1984) identifies "major depression", dysthymia and adjustment disorder with depression in school children. H. Remschmidt (1973) classified circular depression taking into account phenomenological features with separation of lethargic, agitated, hypochondriacal, phobic variants. V.M. Bashina et al. (1999) considered depressive episodes within the 8 most common types of depression in children: adynamic, asthenic, anxious, wistful, melancholic, psychopath-like, dysphoric, somatized, with a group of depressive states, one of the leading symptoms of which was anorectic behavior.

A. A. Severny (1985) noted that only in 14-30% of children the reason for hospitalization were mood disorders, in other cases behavioral disorders, difficulties in learning or psychosomatic disorders were reasons for referral to a psychiatrist. M. Sperling (1959) describes digestive disorders, insomnia, itching, headaches, slow motor skills, tearfulness, lack of interest and a sad appearance as signs of depression in children. In addition, the author believes that the main etiological factor of such conditions is an improper relationship between mother and child (lack of love and understanding). According to many foreign authors (Dugas M., 1966; Annell A., 1969; Schmitz W., 1972; Kuhn V., Kuhn R., 1972), one of the earliest signs of depression is a decrease in school performance. W. Spiel (1961) also believes that diurnal fluctuations of mood in the direction of its decrease in the morning hours of classes deprive the child of compensation and play a decisive role in the occurrence of school phobias. School maladaptation with learning disorder and "school phobia" is one component of "mixed" disorders: a combination of behavioral disorders, depression and suicidal tendencies (Kashani J. H., Simmonds J. P., 1979). J. Puig-Antich (1982) believes that behavioral disorders accompany depression the more often the younger the child is. As the child grows older, aggression, explosive or sexual behavior disappears and passivity increases while the depressive background remains (Poznanski E., Krahenbuhe V., Zrubl J.P. , 1976).

Despite considerable distinctions in views on symptomatology of depression in the child, the majority of authors allocate as its characteristic feature intensity of somatic disorders (Bauersfeld K. H., 1972; Weiberg W. A. et al., 1973; Renshaw D. C., 1974; Kashani J. H. et al., 1981; Kashani J. H., Zababidi Z., 1982; Cheung A. H.; Emslie G. J., Mayes T. L., 2006). Somatic complaints of depression in a child include abdominal pain, chest pain, limb pain, headaches, nausea, and frequent vomiting. In children, a connection between depression and asthma (Pinkerton Ph., 1972), eczema (Altschulova J., 1972), headache (Iovchuk N. M., 1986; Ling W. et al., 1970; Girard J, 1972), and between depression and changes in body weight - obesity or emaciation (Bruch H., 1960; Stadeli H., 1978), depression and pseudoneurological disorders (Maloney M., 1980; Weller R. A. et al., 1991). Comparing psychosomatic symptoms observed in depressed children with similar disorders in adults (based on P. Kielholz, D. Ladewig [1979]), G. Nissen (1970) concludes that only gastrointestinal symptoms are comparable (36 percent in adults, 40 percent in children). Sleep disturbances and headaches were 3 times as common in children, and cardiac pain 16 times as rare as in adults. From the point of view of G. Nissen (1970), in children with depression there is no pain or abnormal sensation in the extremities, hyperhidrosis and respiratory disorders at all, but mutism, nail biting, encopresis and thumb sucking are extremely common.

Attempts to compare depressive conditions in different age groups in parallel also led to the introduction of the term "masked depression" (Glaser K., 1967) in child psychiatry in the late 1960s, similar to the evaluation of atypical depression in adults. Initially, in this application, the term denoted depression in a child that was difficult to recognize because of multiple somatic and behavioral disorders accompanied by negativism, moodiness, grumpiness (Kellner R., Simpson G., Winslow W., 1972).

The term "masked" depression in child psychiatry was first used by K. Glaser (1967, 1981) to describe depression in a child, difficult to recognize because of the abundance of somatic disorders, and depression with negativism,

discontented and grumpy moods   ,

elevated

Sensitivity, asocial and suicidal behavior, which is more typical for teenagers. E. Poznanski, J. P. Zrull (1970), developing diagnostic criteria of depressive disorders in minors, allocated three basic signs: 1) an impression of the child as an unhappy, absent being, complaining that he or she is not loved by anyone and is rejected by loved ones; 2) insomnia; and 3) autoerotic activity of the child. This group quickly expanded, as depression "masked" by a somatic component occurs in 30 % of children - patients of the psychiatric hospital (Anufriev, A. K., 1970; Vertogradova O. P., 1980; Vertogradova O. P. Voloshin V. M., 1989; Sergeyev I. I., Borodin V. I., 1991; Kielholz P., 1972; Nissen G., 1975) and up to 70 % of the depressed patients who address general medical institutions (Isaev D. N.,

1993; Gerish A. A., 1995; Antropov Y. F., 2001).

Later on, the term "masked" depression was increasingly used to refer to "atypical" childhood depression, i.e., not corresponding to the classic clinical picture of "adult" depression. The expansion of the term "masked" depression led to the inclusion of various psychopathological conditions: psychopathic, obsessive-compulsive, anxious-phobic, in addition to somatized ones,

accompanied by reduced affect or concealing it. P. Kielholz (1972) suggested limiting "masked" depressions to those cases of affective pathology in which somatic symptoms come to the fore. More recently, he has drawn a stricter differentiation between larvic depressions and depressive equivalents. In both cases, the depressive symptomatology proper is hidden behind other disorders, but is still recognizable in the first case and almost completely invisible in the second. Many authors (Mamtseva V. N., 1988; Tiganov A. S., 1997; Kellner R. et al., 1972) specify that though somatic and vegetative "masks" of depression are encountered at puberty age, they are more typical for the period of early childhood. However, some believe (Glaser K., 1967) that depression is manifested in a masked form by "somatic" manifestations, mainly in adolescents.

Y.F. Antropov, Y.S. Shevchenko (1999) emphasize that in the structure of morbidity of the child-adolescent population a significant share of mental diseases, in particular those whose main manifestations are somatic disorders and behavioral disorders. These diseases have at their core affective, and in particular depressive disorders and pathology of the instinctive sphere, they are usually qualified as psychosomatic disorders, less often - as somatized (masked) depression and pathological habitual actions. As masks and equivalents of depression in children, according to the authors, most often act as somatic vegetative-visceral disorders, in which disorders of the gastrointestinal tract are often revealed. In middle childhood, there are widespread autonomic-visceral disorders, and in adolescence - functional changes in the cardiovascular system and menstrual disorders in girls. At the same time, according to the authors' observations, somatic disorders are more frequently registered in the structure of anxious depression. Less frequently, depression is masked by behavioral disorders and suicidal behavior.

In the observations of G. Nissen (1973), the most common "psychiatric" symptoms of depression in children were antisociality, anxiety, inhibition, desire for self-isolation, "psychosomatic" symptoms were aggressiveness, enuresis, sleep disorders, mutism and tearfulness. Only in 14 percent of children the reason for hospitalization was a mood disorder; for the rest, behavioral disorders, difficulties in learning and psychosomatic disorders were the reasons for referral to a psychiatrist. J. M. Toolan (962) believes that the older the child, the more depressive feelings prevail over behavioral disorders. Children who have been convinced that they are "unbearable" respond with antisocial behavior that further reinforces feelings of inferiority. They lose their taste for work, have difficulty concentrating, cannot be left alone, seek new stimuli, which leads them to aggressive behavior. The described patterns of depression in children and adolescents by J. M. Toolan (1975) called "depressive equivalents." These terms have since been introduced into child psychiatry to refer to "atypical" depressions.

If Bresser (cited by Nissen G., 1965) believes that depressed children never exhibit criminal tendencies, and B. Frommer (1979) notes in childhood depression anxiety in the indispensable absence of aggression, then M. Dugas (1966), W. von Baeyer (1969), I. Phillips (1979) emphasize the close connection between depressed mood and conduct disorders, including arson, burglary, running away, criminal acts. The frequency of delinquent and antisocial behavior in depressed children is noted by S. Lesse (1974), M. L. Rutter (1976), H. C. Quay (1979), W. Katon et al. (1982), I. T. Dwyer, G. R. Delong (1987), et al. This category, according to the data given by J. Puig-Antich (1982), accounts for 21% of all children and 27% of boys with psychiatric disorders. Glueck et al. (cited by Nissen G., 1972) found behavioral disorders in 14% of depressed children and adolescents, Stoll (cited by Nissen G., 1950) in 50%. In turn, W. A. Weinberg, M. van den Dungen (1972) indicate that in these cases there are clear correlations between depressed mood and poor sociality, lack of tolerance, frustration, loneliness and confusion. M. L. Rutter et al. (1970) suggested that the combination of depressive and behavioral disorders be qualified as "mixed" disorders, M. Kovacs and A. T. Beck (I977) as "complicated".

C. D. Ozeretskovsky (1979), A.E. Lichko (1985) described "delinquent" equivalents of depression, manifested in embitteredness, disobedience, rudeness, propensity to abuse alcohol, drugs. Similar behavioral disorders in depression O. D. Sosiukalo (1984) and V. V. Kovalev (1995) designated as psychopathic equivalents of depression.

Л. S. Yusevich (1946), studying periodic mood disorders (dysphoria) in adolescent offenders with organic lesions of the brain, notes that this type of affective disorders is often found in psychopath-like states. In the clinical picture of "organic dysphoria", the most constant symptom is a wistful mood accompanied by anger, suspicion, hypochondriacal experiences, and delusional ideas. The author, analyzing the dynamics of these disorders, emphasizes that "organic dysphoria" usually develops "gradually," constantly increasing in intensity, accompanied by headaches, a feeling of general weakness and brokenness. Analyzing clinical material, the author assumes that occurrence of "organic dysphoria" is closely connected with changes in vegetative-endocrine system.

In connection with these displays, the child-adolescent affective pathology repeatedly became the subject of study by forensic psychiatrists (T. B. Dmitrieva, 1981; N. B. Morozova, 1986; J. B. Mozhginsky, 1993; V. A. Gurieva, V. A. Gindikin, V. Ya. Y., Semke V. Y., 1994). The revealing of depression in delinquent children and teenagers represents the major problem in view of the high suicide risk (Schaffer D., Greenhill L., 1979; Lesse S., 1980; Marriage K. et al., 1986).

Another widespread variant of pubertal depression was asthenic depression, which is manifested by an unexplained drop in academic performance, intermittent periods of "laziness", boredom and autochthonous episodes of "asthenia" (M.Y. Tsutsulkovskaya, V.A. Mikhailova, 1977; I.V. Oleichik, 1998). C. D. Ozeretskovsky (1979), A.E. Lichko (1985) attributed asthenoapathic disorders and a drop in academic performance to the pubertal age-specific equivalents of the depressive syndrome.

The study of a combination of anxious-phobic, obsessive-compulsive, behavioral, somatoform disorders and depression has defined development of the theory of comorbidity of these disorders (Caron C., Rutter M., 1991). H. M. Van Praag (1998) and a number of other authors (A. B. Smulevich, 1998; I. A. Kozlova, 1999) have emphasized that comorbidity is one of the difficult problems in the study of depression. No matter what positions depression is studied from - biology, epidemiology, therapy - the fact that most patients have a co-morbid diagnosis makes it extremely difficult to interpret scientific data. According to various researchers, comorbidity of depression with other mental disorders in childhood and adolescence is noted in 40-80% of cases (Foa E., Foa U., 1982; Kashani J. H., Carson G. A. et al., 1987; Caron C., Rutter M., 1991; Kovacs M., Devlin B., 1998). However, M. Kovacs (1998) has suggested that comorbidity may be an artifact, reflecting an increase in the number of classification headings of mental disorders and a corresponding intersection of symptoms within and across diagnostic groups. As noted by C. Caron and Rutter (1991), it can be detected if one disorder is a secondary manifestation of a "primary" disorder, or if several disorders are alternative expressions of a single disorder; for example, depression and anxiety are considered alternative manifestations of a single psychopathological process.

The main disorders comorbid with depression are anxiety disorder (20-40%), conduct disorder (8-33%), and obsessive-compulsive disorder (8%). In childhood depression, generalized anxiety disorder and panic disorder are diagnosed in 22% and 14% of cases, respectively. Approximately 18% of patients with panic disorder and 17% of patients with generalized anxiety disorder have depression (Sanderson A., Wetzler G., 1995).

Followers of the American school, who consider mood, anxiety and phobic disorders within the framework of internalized disorders (emotional disorders), confirm the fact that among them there is a high percentage of comorbidity already at the initial stages, which affects the variety of diagnoses established later (Rapee R. M., 1997; Kovacs M., Devlin B., 1998). In children with premorbid anxiety and behavioral disorders, the depressive disorders that develop subsequently reflect the initially found premorbid comorbidity (Rutter M. L., 1981; von Kroff M., Shapiro S. et al., 1987; Torgersen S,, 1990; Rapee R. M., 1997). Comorbidity analysis of major depressive episode and generalized anxiety disorder revealed a common genetic basis for these disorders (Kovacs M., Devlin B., 1998). It has confirmed the opinion of researchers (A. S. Lomachenkov, 1971; O. P. Vertogradova, 1998), who consider anxiety disorders in children and teenagers as a variant of depression.

H. Lehman (1983) states that depression always occurs along with anxiety. The same judgment is held by J. Fawcett, H. Kravitz (1985), who in a group of 200 patients with endogenous depression almost all found different manifestations of anxiety: anxiety - in 72%, somatic symptoms of anxiety - in 42%, a feeling of uncertain threat - in 62%. In these and other works, a close connection of depression and anxiety was found, so close that their clear distinction on psychopathological signs has appeared practically impossible (Nuller J.L., 1988; Breier A., Charney D. S., Heninger G. R., 1985; Kennneth S., Kendler M. D. et al., 1992; Goldstein R. B., Weissman M. M. et al., 1994). At research of chronology of development of anxious and depressive disorders in clinical groups of children and teenagers, it has been found out that in children with the combined anxious and depressive disorders, it was most probable to reveal in premorbid anxious pathology (Savostyanova O.L., 2001; Costello E.J., Costello A.J. et al., 1988). The authors attributed it to the fact that manifestation of depressive disorders is the result of much more complex biological, psychological and cognitive processes, and anxiety is a phylogenetically earlier reaction to a state of discomfort or stress.

No less frequently comorbid with depressive conditions are disorders of behavior. Their combination is noted, according to data of various researchers, in 30-75 % of cases (Bardenstein L.M., Mozhginsky J.B., 2000; van Praag N.M., 1998). The behavioral disorders which are extremely frequent in children during depression fluctuate from elementary anti-disciplinary behaviors to the severe forms of deviant behavior (Sosyukalo O.D., 1984; Tatarova I.N., 1985). Behavioral disorders, as a rule, have a protective character or are caused often by the child's unconscious desire to relieve the state of mind in the company of peers by means of alcohol, smoking, drugs. Many psychiatrists use the term "psychopathic-like depression" to designate depression with behavioral disorders (N.M. Iovchuk, 1989; I.A. Kozlova, 1999; A.S. Kurashov, 2001).

Л. M. Bardenstein (2000) points out that "psychopathic" and "psychopath-like" conditions are similar in a number of external manifestations, but have different bases. Unlike psychopathic syndromes which represent manifestations of personality abnormalities, in psychopathoid disorders, signs of an ongoing disease process or consequences of brain trauma come to the fore. Vroneau (1989) also believed that psychopathology-like disorders are based on such factors as "an ongoing process of endogenous structure or organic nature, residual phenomena of an endogenous process or organic CNS lesion. It is these factors that cause essential differences from similar disorders in neuroses and psychopathies".

Thus, the term "psychopath-like" depression should be understood to mean states in which signs similar in a number of external manifestations to psychopathic states are caused by a depressive disorder. This approach inevitably raises the question of developing differential-diagnostic criteria for states whose clinical picture simultaneously exhibits both depressive symptoms and psychopathic symptoms (Ozeretsky N.I., 1938; Kurashov A.S., 2001). The differential diagnosis assumes division of three similar in the clinical picture, but different in essence conditions: 1) the occurrence of depression in a psychopath; 2) the intensification of character accentuations with the occurrence of a depressive episode; and 3) the appearance of behavioral reactions not previously characteristic of the personality against the background of depression. The anamnestic approach is basic for the primary division.

There are other approaches to the study of depressive states with behavioral disorders. N. M. Iovchuk (1989) divided psychopathic-like depressions into two variants of depressive states according to the type of a leading affect - dysphoric depressions and the so-called Unlust-depressions. The main differences of these two groups were the presence of accessory symptoms in Unlust-depression, ideas of unjust attitude with a predominant limitation of aggression to the family circle, suicidal behavior, which could be explained by the influence of endogenous process, since Unlust-depression was mainly observed in the schizophrenia structure.

M. Sh. Vroneau (1971) noted, that in childhood, there are seldom the states exhausted by the symptoms obligatory for depression, more often there are polymorphic pictures. However, difficulty in diagnosis is caused not only by polymorphism, but also by isomorphism of clinical manifestations, i.e. external similarity at different essence, which is especially expressed at an adolescent age.

T. F. Papadopoulos (1983) describes 5 stages of depression in adults: dysthymic-dysbolic, cyclothymic, melancholic, delusional, paraphrenic. The first is the mildest stage of a depressive episode. Morbid disorders are limited to somatovegetative disturbances and changes in well-being in the form of a peculiar decrease in the general tone with asthenic phenomena. One of the first signs is sleep disturbance. Appetite decreases, tendency to constipation is manifested, sensations of bodily discomfort, hyperesthesia and tearfulness are expressed. Decreased tone is characterized by patients as lethargy, laziness, apathy, impotence, and powerlessness. Clinically important is the close association of well-being with the diurnal rhythm. The cyclothymic stage is characterized by the accession of differentiated feelings of longing, depression, vague anxiety, pessimistic orientation of thinking, i.e. typical symptoms are pronounced affective disorders, weakening of vital stimuli on the background of somatotropic disturbances.

Similar descriptions of childhood and teenage depression are found in many authors (N.M. Iovchuk, 1989; V. Kovalev. V., 1995; Antropov Y. F., Shevchenko Y. S., 1999; Bashina V. M., 1999; Nissen G., 1972). They allocate typical signs of the children's endogenous depression: massiveness of somatoalgic and behavioral disorders, fragmentariness, change of character and degree of expressiveness of the affective component, variety of shades of the pathological affect with prevalence of anxiety or dysphoria, frequency of episodes of psychomotor agitation with the rich atypical affect. At the same time, the authors believe that the signs characteristic of "adult" depression often look unimpressive. Nevertheless, purposeful examination of the patient can reveal a depressed state, high physical and mental fatigue, increased irritability, and the presence of, although subdued, but often detectable daily variations of well-being and mood.

From our point of view, the specified clinical picture corresponds to the first and second stages of development of a depressive attack described in adults by T. F. Papadopoulos (1983). The melancholic stage in adolescents is described less often, and delirium and paraphrenia are described in general in isolated cases and only in the structure of schizophrenia (Danilova L.Yu., 1985; Kozlova I.A., 1999; Wieck Ch., 1965; Bender L., 1966). In other words, depression in childhood differs from depression in adults rather quantitatively than qualitatively. Differences in the formulation of complaints of depression in different age groups are connected in many respects with the ability of adults to analyze and verbalize their feelings and the insufficiency of such abilities in adolescents (Shaffer D., 1996; Nissen G., 1972; Kandel D., Davies M., 1986). But even adults have difficulties in describing painful experiences due to the strangeness of sensations, which causes them to resort to metaphorical description (Vrono M. Sh., 1971; Nuller Y. L., 1988). Despite the difference in the description of painful sensations of adults and adolescents, the analysis of complaints reveals a clear enough analogy between them. If adults describe melancholy as "heaviness, a stone in the chest," "loss of the meaning of life, joy," "collapse of life" and at the same time distinguish these conditions from the experience of grief experienced with various misfortunes, children complain about "boredom," "sadness," desire to cry, besides not being able to compare these sensations. It is necessary to notice that the description of "heaviness in the chest" becomes a quite widespread complaint at children's age (V.N. Mamtseva, 1982; N.M. Iovchuk, 1989).

G. Nissen (1980, 1981, 1982, 1984) includes in the nosological systematics of childhood depression. Nissen (1980, 1981, 1982, 1984) includes, in addition to endogenous, reactive-neurotic and somatogenic (exogenous, symptomatic) depression, playing "an absolutely dominant role" in childhood. Somatogenic depressions are sometimes found from birth, often characterized by a chronic course, and the psychogenic ones - after 5 years of age. Somatogenic depressions are a consequence of a cerebral organic lesion, while reactive ones are a "motivated response" to mental trauma, due to a disorder of the central mental regulatory mechanism due to a genetic predisposition or an acquired particular personality disposition.

Suicides occupy a special place in the clinic of depressive disorders in children. Suicide in pediatric practice has long ceased to be perceived as a casuistic case. Considering children's suicidal actions, it is necessary to take into account that the concept of death as a category of termination of life, as a rule, has not been formed in them yet. Thus, suicides of a child and an adult are fundamentally different. Up to the age of 3, the child does not yet have borders separating him or her from the outside world and does not distinguish between the categories "alive" and "dead". As a rule, preschool children have already formed some ideas of death. Nevertheless, they often consider death to be solely the fate of old people and do not allow for the idea of ending one's own life. Besides, most children of this age lack understanding of the irreversibility of death. Schoolchildren already have a clear distinction between the concepts of life and death, even though death is still viewed as a temporary phenomenon. Almost all girls from the age of 12 years and boys from the age of 15 years understand the finality of their own life and worry about it, but only 20% of teenagers are aware that death is the final termination of physical and spiritual life (Isaev D.N., 1993). However among the causes of death of children and teenagers suicide takes the second place, being second only to cardiovascular diseases (Larsson B., Melin L., 1992).

In an anonymous survey of Swedish adolescents, 3-6% of the respondents have ever attempted suicide (Gillberg K., Hellgren L., 2004), and few of them have seen a doctor. In recent years the number of suicides in this age group continues to increase. A. V. Golenkov, A. B. Kozlov, T. V. Tsurupa, S. V. Pavlov (1998) in studying suicides among children and teenagers in Chuvashia revealed a 66.8% increase in completed suicides among children and teenagers in 1997 as compared to 1993: from 8.88 per 100,000 of the corresponding age population to 14.81. The suicide rate among adolescents averaged 24.07 per 100,000 of the population of corresponding age, while among children it was only 1.76 (among children and adolescents the average was 8.63 per 100,000 of the population). Thus, boys are almost three times more likely to commit suicide than girls; children and adolescents living in rural areas are 1.5-1.7 times more likely than their urban counterparts, respectively. The works of A. I. Lazebnik (1998, 2000) in the Udmurt Republic testify to the increase of suicidal tendencies.

Among the basic risk factors of suicide of children it is possible to allocate genetic (McHolm A. E., 2004), ethno-cultural (Runeson B., 1992), mental, family (Maris R. M., 1981; Miller K., King C., Shain B., Naylor M., 1992; Pfeffer C. R., Normadin L., Kakuma T., 1998). Suicide of parents or relatives can be a peculiar example of how the person "solves" problems (Fredman R. C., 1984).

Until now, however, the factor of mental health is of the greatest importance. Even Esquirol considered that all suicides are mentally ill, as only in a state of insanity a person can attempt his life (Esquirol A. L., 1838). Further this opinion was confirmed by many researchers, V.J. Gindikin gave data, according to which in 90 % of cases true suicidal behavior occurs with psychotic states, and A.L. Berman's researches have revealed that people suffering from ^diagnosed mental disorders commit about 90 % of suicides (V.V. Kovaleva, 1981). The same tendencies are revealed in children and teenagers.

According to research of Swedish, Finnish and American scientists of suicides among children by psychological autopsy, psychiatric diagnoses are determined in 91-98% of the subjects (Runeson B., 1989; Rich C. L., Sherman M., Fowler R. C., 1990; Marttunen M. D., Henrikson M. M. et al., 1991; Brent D. A., Perper J. A., Moritz G., Allman C. et al., 1993, Shaffer D., Fisher P., Trautman P. et al., 2006). Finnish children who committed suicide were mostly diagnosed with depression or "adjustment disorder" (Runeson B., 1992). In a large American study of young people who died by suicide before age 20, depression was a common diagnosis before age 17 (Shaffer D., Fisher P., Trautman P. et al., 2006).

Presented studies determine that one of the leading causes of suicide among children is depressive mood disorders (Shaffer D., Fisher P., Trautman P. et. al., 1996; Goldstein T. R., Birmaher B., Axelson D. et al., 2005; Barbe R. P., Williamson D. E., Bridge J. A., 2005; Wasserman G. A., 2006). Thus, according to a study by T. R. Goldstein (2005), among 450 children with a major depressive episode, one-third of those examined had a suicidal history. O. Shiryaev, A. Neretina, G. Kosheleva (2006), studying 132 cases of childhood suicide attempts, revealed a depressive mood disorder in the majority of the sample.

A. Schopenhauer, the creator of the pessimistic philosophy that became widespread in Europe from the second half of the 19th century, said that he who commits suicide actually wants to live. He is merely dissatisfied with the conditions in which he exists. This statement essentially actualizes the problem of early diagnosis and treatment of depressive mood disorders among children.

Most psychiatrists believe that depressive disorders are a frequent component of many mental illnesses, affecting their essence and structure, and that early identification of the nosological identity of the disorder is necessary to determine prognosis and therapeutic approaches (Vrono M. Sh., 1979; Kovalev V. V., 1979; Tiganov A. S., Vidmanova L. N., Platonova T. P.,Suhonsky A. A., 1986; Mosolov S. N., 1995; Panteleeva G. P., 1999; Nissen G., 1972).

The authors who share this opinion, when studying depression in adulthood, adolescence, adolescence and childhood, use the most traditional classification of P. Kielholz (1972), which is based on the nosological principle.

It distinguishes organic, symptomatic, schizophrenic, cyclical, neurotic and reactive depression. In domestic psychiatry, the approaches to the study of adult and child affective pathology largely coincide. In adults and adolescents, depressive states are described within schizophrenia, including schizoaffective psychoses, manic-depressive psychosis; neurotic disorders, reactive states, as well as in the structure of psychopathic personality development (Snezhnevsky A. V., 1968; Tsutsulkovskaya M. J., Panteleeva G. P., 1986; Vertogradova O. P., Voloshin V. M., 1989; Tiganov, A. S., 1997; Smulevich, A. B., 1997). The psychiatrists studying depressive conditions in childhood and adolescence allocate the same nosological categories (Vrono M. Sh., 1971; Mamtseva V. N., 1982; Danilova L. Y., 1986; Kovalev V. V., 1995; Bashina V. M., 1999; Kozlova I. A., 1999), and a distinctive feature of childhood and adult age is the different specific weight of their clinical manifestations in these nosological groups.

The study of affective pathology in this context is fraught with great difficulties, foremost among which is the lack of conceptual unity in the views on the formation of these disorders in children and, consequently, the absence of a unified correct clinical classification and typology that takes into account the frequently encountered signs of psychiatric dysontogenesis. Of the multitude of interpretations of the psychopathological essence of affective disorders in childhood, three main ones can be distinguished.

The clinico-nosological trend recognizes the presence of childhood depression and attempts to describe its psychopathological features in terms similar to those of mature affective disorders. Another group of psychiatrists argue in favor of the presence of predominantly masked depressions in childhood, which are interpreted very broadly, up to including bedwetting, socialization disorders, school failure, phobias, and other disorders. Representatives of psychoanalytical concepts of psychoses either deny the possibility of formation of early depression because of underdevelopment of the "superego" in children, or point to the formation of special phobic, encompassing, uretic conditions, without attributing the latter to actually depressive (Dmitrieva T.B., Makushkin

E.V., Fedina M.A., 2001).

1.4.1 Peculiarities of the course of the depressive syndrome in children with schizophrenia

Г. G.F. Kolotilin (1971) attributed to the cardinal diagnostic signs of depression in schizophrenia, besides monotony of affect, pretentiousness and inadequacy of suicidal actions, presence of delirium-like fantasizing with elements of pseudo-hallucinations and ideas of influence. W. Spiel (1961) considered the features of schizophrenic depressions to be empty affect, the predominance in the clinical picture of apathy, fatigue, lethargy, sometimes combined with confusion and anxiety.

A significant contribution to the study of child and adolescent affective pathology in the structure of individual nosologies has been made by domestic psychiatrists. N.M. Iovchuk (1976, 1981, 1989), studying in his works affective disorders in childhood schizophrenia, concludes that these disorders can arise in any age period of childhood in psychopathologically peculiar forms. The author identifies the following features of endogenous depressions in children: massiveness of somatoalgic and behavioral disorders, masking affective symptoms; multidimensional shades of pathological affect; smoothness of the daily rhythm of affect; fragmentarity, variability of character and degree of intensity of disorders; frequency of episodes of psychomotor agitation with intense atypical affect and somatovegetative crises. Age dynamics of the depressive syndrome, according to the researcher, consists in transition from somato-vegetative and pseudo-aggressive manifestations predominating in infancy to predominantly neurosis-like at younger preschool age with accession of somatoalgic and rudimentary delirium at older preschool age, their increase in combination with massive ideational and abulic disorders at a younger school age and in manifestation of distinct depressive ideas, behavioral and characteristic pubertal disorders in prepubertal age.

B. M. Bashina (1981) developed a typology of affective disorders in various forms of the childhood schizophrenic process. Thus, in the structure of attack-like schizophrenia with a low-progressive course 6 types of depression were singled out: asthenic, simple bitchy, moody (grumpy), with marked senestoalgic manifestations, with disorders of self-consciousness, agitated. On the basis of the research, the author concludes that a specific type of affective disorders corresponds to different forms of childhood schizophrenia.

Г. Е. Sukhareva (1955) referred to "loss of freshness of vital affect", increased protopathic emotionality with the appearance of unmotivated anxiety, fear and disappearance of feelings of sympathy for loved ones as symptoms characteristic of schizophrenia in its early stages. She pointed to the need to identify subtle disorders, primarily thought disorders, which were of greater diagnostic value than psychotic symptoms. A. S. Lomachenkov (1971) described affective disorders in schizophrenia as combined with emotional and mental inadequacy, ideatorial-motor dissociation, tension, paradoxicality and unmotivation.

С. Д. Ozeretskovsky (1988), who studied the initial manifestations of manic-depressive psychosis and schizophrenia with affective disorders in adolescents, pointed out that manic-depressive psychosis is rare in pubertal age and noted a number of features of schizophrenic depression, to which he referred a smaller degree than in cyclothymic depression, The author noted a number of specific features of schizophrenic depression, including less pronounced somatic complaints, presence of schizophrenic psychosis precursors in the form of abortive psychosensory disorders, transient states of confusion with troubling confusion of thoughts, accession of unmotivated fear, depersonalizing and obsessive experiences, thought disorders with intrusions, interruptions of thoughts and resonance. The author considered the increasing polymorphism of affective seizures to be the most specific feature in favor of schizophrenia. Additional features not peculiar to manic-depressive psychosis in adolescents included fear and absence of self-blaming ideas about depression. G.P. Panteleeva, M.Y. Tsutsulkovskaya (1986) give descriptions of dysphoric moody erased depressions in the initial state of malignant schizophrenia, protracted "stupid", adynamic and acute polymorphic anxious depressions as part of a manifest attack in circular and schuboid schizophrenia, as well as protracted polymorphic states with predominance of predominantly pubertal disorders (dysmorphobic, depersanalizing, heboid, supersensory). The variants of masked depressions in childhood schizophrenia are of particular importance in children's clinics. I. N. Tatarova (1985), O. D. Sosyukalo (1984), A. A. Severny (1992) describe cases of hyperthermia, vegetovascular disorders and behavioral disorders as "masks".

The division into types of depressive conditions among children proposed by N.M. Iovchuk, A.A. Severny (1999) is based on the definition of a leading disorder that dominates over other depressive symptomatology and does not disappear during periods of its temporary weakening: the character of the prevailing mood, and in the absence of its differentiation and stability - ideational, motor or somatovegetative disorders. Taking into account the features of the clinical picture, 14 variants of depression in childhood have been described.

1. Simple depression is characterized by an undifferentiated lowered mood with the predominance of sadness and grief, accompanied by lowered self-esteem and a pessimistic assessment of the present and future, without significant motor and ideatorial lethargy.

2. Mopey depression is characterized by a combination of melancholic affect with ideational and motor retardation, depressive delusions of self-blame and self-deprecation.

3. Feelings of internal tension, uneasiness, unreasonable, meaningless anxiety are typical for anxious depression, in which anxious fears of a concrete nature are noted at times.

4. The fearful depressive state proceeds with the predominant affect of fear. Fear on the background of depression acts as a characteristic disorder of childhood, a universal form of reaction that appears in a exaggerated form and gives depression as a whole a fearful connotation.

5. The tearful form of a depressive condition is characterized by crying abundantly, arising for any insignificant reason or without reason. Crying has a character of almost constant whimpering, whining, capriciousness, or readiness to cry with occasional prolonged sobbing, wailing and screaming. At the same time, there are no complaints about a decrease in mood, or the young child cannot express them. Tearfulness appears in combination with sleep disturbance, loss of appetite, complaints of boredom and unpleasant bodily sensations or pains in various parts of the body.

6. Dysphoric depression is characterized by the prevalence of atypical malevolent affect with dissatisfaction with others   , irritability, irascibility, irascibility, sometimes leading to outbursts of rage and aggression with a desire to destroy.

7. Stuporotic depression is characterized by an extreme degree of motor and ideational retardation, at times reaching a state of complete immobility with weakness or lack of response to the environment, cessation of verbal contact, refusal of food and a temporary suspension or even regression of behavior and skills. Affective disorders proper in these cases are mainly anxiety or fear, the presence of which becomes obvious when stupor disorders alternate with psychomotor agitation or only after the appearance of contact with the patient when the depressive state weakens.

8. Depression with psychopath-like disorders is considered as a depressive state in which disorders mimicking character pathology (rudeness, insolence, spitefulness, aggressiveness, oppositionality, hyperexcitability, despotism, hysteroidism, etc.), act in conjunction with behavioral disorders: truancy, refusal to attend school, fighting, anti-disciplinary behaviors, abandonment, vagrancy, substance use, early sexual intercourse, and sometimes criminal actions. Behavioral disorders, which extremely often occur during depression in prepubertal children and adolescents and mask it, range from elementary anti-disciplinary behaviors to severe forms of deviant behavior.

9. Adynamic depression is a depressive condition in which energy

disorders are in the foreground: reduction of impulses, impotence, lethargy, laziness, weakness of the emotional response with subjective weakness of the feeling of lowered mood. In the mildest cases, adynamic depression is limited to complaints of constant weariness, fatigue, unwillingness to engage in activities and even play, and a dulling of interests. Adynamic depression is accompanied by sluggishness and inactivity, although ideational and motor lethargy are absent or minimal.

10. Fatigability, exhaustion, irritability and hyperaesthesia (intolerance of bright light, loud sounds) are in the foreground in asthenic-like depression, in this connection, the depressive condition has a certain similarity to the asthenic syndrome. In asthenic-like depression, patients primarily complain of lethargy, weakness, fatigue, intolerance of school work, noise, bright lights, resentfulness, tearfulness, headaches, heaviness throughout the body, unpleasant bodily sensations, general malaise, memory loss. Fatigue, fatigue, impaired memory and concentration are, however, not truly asthenic, appearing already at the beginning of work and being replaced by increased work capacity at the end of the day.

11. Stupid depression is a depressive condition in which ideatorial lethargy predominates in the absence or weak expression of inhibition in the sphere of motor skills and a depressive mood is erased. Schoolchildren with this type of depression have a sharp drop in learning, connected with loss of ability to perceive new information, a subjective sensation of memory loss, difficulty to reproduce new material and to concentrate attention. At the expressed and long term character of stupid depression, there is the so-called depressive pseudo-debility imitating oligophrenia. Against this background, there are unexpressed ideas of inadequacy, self-deprecation, sensitized ideas of attitude, fear of school, sometimes with a complete refusal of attending it, accompanied by bouts of crying, hysterical reactions or dysphoric episodes with anger, aggression and destructive tendencies.

12. Anesthetic depression is a depressive state, proceeding with the prevalence of anaesthesia psychica dolorosa - mental anesthesia, a sense of

painful insensitivity, characterized by the loss of feelings, including love for loved ones, joy, sadness, horror, the disappearance of the possibility of empathy, compassion, emotional resonance, accompanied by painful experience of his emotional change. Anesthetic depression occurs infrequently and only from adolescence onward, has a protracted character and most often proceeds with little or no painful component of mental anesthesia.

13. Somatized depression is a depressive symptom-complex in which one or another, low-symptomatic or polymorphic, somatovegetative symptomatology comes to the fore, imitating primary somatic pathology, masking, hiding actual depressive manifestations, which, nevertheless, are always present and can be detected.

14. "Juvenile asthenic incompetence"-the fundamental disorder in these cases is an inability to concentrate thoughts, a distractibility unrelated to external circumstances and at the same time not caused by the presence of dominant thought displacing actual perception and assimilation. This disorder is involuntary and uncontrollable; extraneous thoughts are sometimes perceived as violent intrusions. The next most frequent symptom of ideational disorder is difficulty understanding meaning. Listening or reading, the teenager understands only separate words, phrases, but cannot catch their logical relationship and, accordingly, understand the whole, i.e. there is a violation of the higher cognitive synthesis. Less often there are "small ideatorial automatisms" such as "breaks" of thoughts, "switching off" of thoughts, parallel, chaotic and intertwined thoughts up to a complete inability to communicate verbally.

1.4.2. Depressive syndrome in children with neurotic disorders

Speaking about affective pathology of children and teenagers, it is impossible to ignore the group of psychogenic disorders in which structure depression is rather frequent clinical manifestation. T.B. Dmitrieva (1980, 1981), studying psychogenic depression in adolescents, noted the originality of affective manifestations during puberty: a significant intensity of vegetative-vascular and neurotic disorders, neurotic level of disorganization of mental activity, atypicality of the depressive symptoms proper, inclusion of specific teenage behavioral reactions in the clinical picture. H. Remschmidt et al. (1973) and Ch. Eggers (1980, 1981) differentiate reactive depression from neurotic depression in children. Reactive depression is extremely frequent in childhood, runs with a decrease in the general vital tone, sleep disorders, appetite, paroxysms of anxiety and is caused by acute mental trauma, removal from the family or violation of the relationship between the child and his or her parents. Neurotic depression caused by a chronic conflict situation is expressed in the "chronic syndrome of helplessness (or abandonment)" with bouts of crying, agitation, withdrawal, sleep disorders, anorexia, enuresis, encopresis. The most outlined reactive depression in adolescents is described by forensic psychiatrists (Natalevich E.S., Koroleva V.D. et al., 1982).

From the variety of clinical variants of reactive depression existing in psychiatric practice, the authors allocate the following in adolescents: asthenic, anxious, dysphoric, hysterical, and hypochondriac. Within the framework of psychogenic depressions of childhood R. Spitz (1946) describes "anaclitic depression" which develops in infants as a result of their isolation from their mother. V.A. Gurieva (1996) observed rather frequent cases of the so-called sibling depressions in children during the period of 2.5-5 years, arising after the birth of the second child. The author noted that it was especially pronounced in children who were brought up as "family idols", "spoiled" or characterized by personality abnormality.

On the basis of clinical and psychopathological features on the basis of the accompanying affective manifestations of hypothymia, Y.F. Antropov (2001) allocated the following typological variants of neurotic depression. 1. The anxious variant with a lowered mood, anxiety, a feeling of internal tension, sometimes with inability to carry out purposeful activity. Children are restless, with chaotic motor activity, with anxiety about life, fear of death, fear for the life of close relatives. 2. The asthenic variant is characterized by lethargy, low activity, fatigue, unwillingness to do anything, increased fatigability and intolerance of mental tension. 3. The asthenic-anxious variant of neurotic depression concerns polymorphic variants including other (asthenia, anxiety), not expressed affective displays along with hypothymia. This variant includes, along with unexpressed affect of longing, asthenic, anxious and vegetovisceral manifestations. 4. Anxiety and melancholy variant proceeds with expressed anxiety and melancholy in combination with vegetovisceral disorders and rudimentary hysterical and hypochondriacal disorders.

1.4.3. Depressive syndrome in children with mental retardation

Episodic and recurrent psychoses in oligophrenia are described by many domestic (Felinskaya N. I., 1950; Freyerov O. E., 1964; Kovalev V. V., 1995) and foreign authors (Ellis N. R., 1982; Bortnick-Duffy S. A., 1990). The majority of authors consider these psychoses as specific for the mentally retarded. Their clinical picture and course differ from other forms of mental diseases (schizophrenia, circular psychosis, exogenous psychoses) which can develop on the basis of mental retardation. Psychoses of this group have been described by various authors under different names: "psychoses in oligophrenics," "psychoses in retardation," "amorphous psychoses," etc. Their occurrence at pubertal and adolescent ages is underlined (G. E. Sukhareva, 1965, O.D. Sosyukalo, 1966).

The etiology and pathogenesis of psychoses in oligophrenics are still not clear enough. The role of vascular and liquor-dynamic disorders is assumed. The occurrence of psychoses during the transitional phase of development, most often during puberty, suggests a pathogenetic role of a dysharmonious pubertal crisis. Although psychoses often start due to the influence of external factors (psychogenic or exogenic-organic), it is not always possible to note symptoms typical of psychogenic or infectious psychoses in the clinical picture of the disease. Pathogenetic mechanisms specific to this or that form can also play a certain role in the development of psychoses. An increased frequency of psychoses with subsequent regression of mental functions in adults and teenagers with Down's disease has been observed (Burelov E.A., 1980; Gurieva V.A., 1995,

1996).

The manifestation of psychosis in oligophrenics is atypical both in clinic and in course. The basic symptomatology of oligophrenia is quite brightly revealed both in the content of psychotic experiences and in a certain specificity of the psychopathological syndromes themselves. It is characterized by poverty and elementary psychopathological manifestations. In many patients, somatoneurological signs are noted in the clinical structure of psychosis: headache, dizziness, sleep disorder, acute fatigue and exhaustion, change of alertness levels of consciousness.

A common feature of psychoses in oligophrenics is their episodic character. At the end of the psychosis, the patient's condition usually returns to the initial state. In a number of cases, a relapsing course is observed, with clear alternation of psychotic states with complete recovery. An attack lasts 1 to 2 weeks. Light intervals between psychotic attacks usually last from 2 to 3 to 4 weeks. Asthenic manifestations with headache, increased excitability and irritability, hypertension occur during the interictal periods.

Psychoses with predominance of affective disorders most often present in the form of dysphoric and depressive states. Dysphoric psychoses are manifested by mood disorders of a melancholic tone, irritability, propensity to aggressive actions. During these periods, patients are tense, negativistic and quite often experience fear and anxiety. Severe headaches, dizziness and sleep disorders are noted. At the expressed dysphoric condition, a short-term disorder of consciousness by type of crepuscular with the subsequent amnesia of this period can be observed (Vvedensky I. N., 1940; Beier D. C., 1964; Ellis N. R., 1982).

Depressive states are usually superficial, are characterized by a monotonous lowered mood with a dysphoric or dysthymic edge. Often depressive episodes are accompanied by anxiety, undifferentiated fears and nervousness and confusion. Some teenagers with shallow intellectual defects reveal unstable, unformed ideas of attitude and self-blaming: such patients consider themselves "bad", "fools", they feel that people look at them, "want to jinx", sometimes suicidal behavior is possible (O.E. Freyerov, 1964; G.E. Sukhareva, 1965; V.V. Gorinov, 1986; N. Dzeruzhinskaya. A., 1994; Berezantsev A. Yu., 1991; Gurieva V.A., 1996). The abundance of hypochondriacal expressions and senestopathies is characteristic. Hypochondriac complaints of patients are characterized by polymorphism, variability, fluctuations of intensity and pathological sensations. Their content is simple, primitive, concrete, often accompanied by seeking help from others, with no delusional interpretation of pathological sensations. The complaints are presented by the patients in the form of obtrusive clinging, lamentations (Vvedensky I.N., 1940; Petrov L.A., 1960; Gorinov V.V., 1989; Kovalev V.V., 1995).

1.4.4. Peculiarities of the course of the depressive syndrome in children against the background of of residual organic lesions of the central nervous system

Drawing an analogy between "chronic" depression and the hyperkinetic syndrome in children, H. Stadeli (1978) suggested that minimal cerebral dysfunction underlies these two disorders. The connection of depression in childhood with minimal cerebral dysfunction (MMD) is also noted by W. Schmitz (1972) E. Puzynska, M. Mazurzak (1978), D. A. Waller, J. A. Ruch (1983), I. Kolvin et al. (1984) consider MMD a necessary substrate of depression and reject depression of other genesis in childhood. C. J. Kestenbaum (1979) believes that MMD leads to the early development of affective phases, and that manic-depressive psychosis in adults has the same nature but it is less obvious, and sees a genetic predisposition in families with manic-depressive psychosis in the inheritance of MMD.

According to G. Gollnitz (1972), depressive states in children have no direct connection with cerebral insufficiency, but have it indirectly in the form of secondary reactive depression. According to R. Corboz (1972), depression in children with psychorganic syndrome is rare and is a reaction to learning difficulties, parental cruelty. Children with a particularly differentiated mental structure and high intelligence are significantly more likely to exhibit depressive reactions than children with cerebral insufficiency.

However, there is now evidence that fetal injuries, birth trauma and other injuries that lead to the formation of a psychorganic syndrome also have a higher risk of developing depressive disorders (Gillberg K., Hellgren L., 2004). Depressive-dysthymic neurosis-like conditions are disorders of the neurotic level of response that arise in connection with cerebral disturbances, which are caused by residual-organic disorders of the brain. According to V.S. Aleshko (1970), V.V. Kovalev (1995), these states have age differences. In children of preschool and younger school age, the lowered mood is combined with caprice, propensity to monotonous crying, quite often with vague fears. At high school age, a more expressed depressive affect in combination with anxiety, hypochondriacal fears, irritability and dissatisfaction is noted. Adolescents occasionally have thoughts about their own worthlessness and the uselessness of life. Often, especially with consequences of brain infections, depressive-dysthymic conditions are accompanied by episodic disorders of sensory synthesis. There are various vegetative disorders (hyperhidrosis, absence of appetite, vasovagal disorders), sleep disorders. In the form of episodic disorders in combination with other neurosis-like disorders, depressive-dysthymic disorders occur quite often (V. V. Kovalev, 1995).

CHAPTER II.
ONTOGENESIS OF DEPRESSIVE SYMPTOMS IN CHILDHOOD

Different ages of the child have different significance for the occurrence of various mental disorders, but the period of psychobiological development, which is childhood, is the most vulnerable in this respect. Mental development in children in general occurs unevenly, but in certain periods it also becomes disharmonious, when formation of some functions lags behind others or, on the contrary, outpaces them (Gurieva V.A., Dmitrieva T.B., Makushkin E.V. et al., 2007). According to V. A. Gurieva (2001), in the child-adolescent psychiatry, the idea of dynamics acquires a special meaning. The question is not only about clinical formation of this or that pathological condition, but also that any mental illness proceeds against a background of an ongoing psychobiological state which, on the one hand, is broken under the influence of the disease process (Osipova E.A., 1940) and on the other - defines resources of reacting psyche, influencing clinical design of a psychopathological condition. Discovery of clear clinical and age-specific regularities of occurrence and development of mental diseases and pathological conditions, as well as social problems characteristic of each age, determined the separation of two disciplines: child and adolescent psychiatry. It was substantiated about 130 years ago by G. Maudsley (1870) "the idea of development", which formed the basis of "developmental psychology", "developmental psychiatry" and "ontogenesis".

Ontogenesis is understood as the process of individual development of an organism, which is a set of regular, interrelated, consecutive morphological, physiological and metabolic transformations in the organism from the moment of its isolation as an individual (in humans from the fusion of germ cells of parents) to death. Ontogenesis is divided into embryonic (germinal, perinatal), lasting from fertilization to birth (in humans it is divided into embryonic proper - the first 7 weeks of development, and fetal, ending with childbirth) and postembryonic (postnatal) periods. According to the unified biogenetic law (Haeckel E., 1866), ontogenesis is a brief and concise repetition of phylogenesis - the process of historical development of individual types, classes, families, genera, species of living organisms.

The influence of ontogenesis on mental disorders is multidimensional. Firstly, practically all psychopathological symptoms, syndromes and diseases at different age periods (youth, adulthood and old age) proceed differently, and this is the expediency of separating child psychiatry, adolescent psychiatry and gerontopsychiatry into separate blocks. For example, asthenic and depressive syndromes, hypochondriac and paranoid syndromes, without losing their basic phenomenological essence, will manifest themselves quite differently and have their specificity at different stages of ontogenesis.

Secondly, although there is still no exhaustive information on the role of the age factor, there are studies which show that various stress factors and situations have a psychotraumatic influence at various stages of ontogenesis and that those of them which have no psychotraumatic influence at a certain stage of ontogenesis can already become pathogenic or sanogenic at the following stage (V.V. Semke, 1989; N.A. Smulevich, 1989). For children, for example, leading psychogenic factors of neuroticization are disorders of family relations, unfavorable influences from parents, impairment of the need to be, the need to express oneself, the need for support, love and recognition, undeserved punishments, parents' divorce, etc. (Zakharov, 1982).

The sudden emotional rejection by loved ones to whom the adolescent has great affection or the news that he or she is an adopted child (Lichko A.E., 1985) is especially difficult to endure. In young and average age, family, domestic and service conflicts, fear for the life and physical well-being and sexual problems come to the fore. Psychogenias of late age present a different picture. Most often, the psychologically traumatic factor is illness and death of close people, fear of one's own illness and death, fear of growing old and retirement. These reasons are so widespread that there are even terms "pension illness" and "pension bankruptcy" (Averbukh E. S., Teleshevskaya M. E., 1976).

Thirdly, it is noticed that some syndromes have a certain age tropism. Despite the similarity of psychologically traumatic influences, the personality reacts to them differently and with different symptomatology depending on what stage of ontogenesis it is at. And in the process of ontogenesis itself, it is possible to observe a transformation of symptomatology in the same person under the influence of the same psychologically traumatic situation when conducting a longitudinal study.

Research of leading gerontologists in our country (Averbukh E. S., Teleshevskaya M. E., 1976; Semke V. V., Odarchenko S. S., 2006) have shown that neurotic pictures in late age, in particular neurasthenia, are characterized by less dynamic, motley and diverse symptomatology. Hysterical neuroses are observed less and less often with age. They are superseded by asthenic, neurasthenic symptomatology combined with anxious-phobic, depressive and hypochondriac symptoms. Recent research of age-specific features of neuroses and neurotic syndromes (Grineva I. M., Hoholeva A. A., 1989) have shown, that obsessive-phobic and hypochondriacal symptoms are more typical for patients with early onset of disease (up to age 20-25), while asthenic and depressive symptoms are typical for late-onset patients (after age 25). Thus, a single multidimensional scheme of the influence of psychotraumatic

факторов на личность, представленная В. Я. Семке (2006) и характеризующая непрерывное и взаимосвязанное патогенетическое влияние на индивид в процессе его жизненного пути (рис. 1).

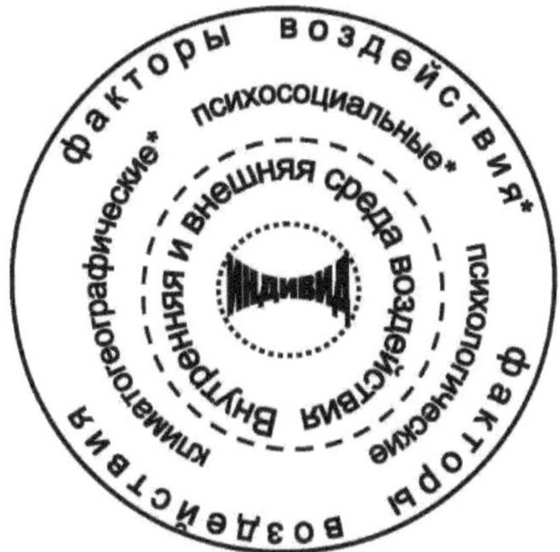

Рис. 1. Факторы патогенетического и саногетического влияния на личность человека в процессе онтогенеза

Generalizing the data of various authors (Vygotsky L. S., 1960; Sukhareva G. E., 1974; Garbuzov V. I., 1980; Lichko A. E., 1985; Serdyukovskaya G. N., 1985; Buhler Ch., 1931; Gessel A., 1956; Desunis G., 1962), who studied the mental development of the child at early stages of ontogenesis, it is possible to allocate the following stages which have the basic value in child development.

In the first year of life, the child focuses on reducing the psycho-physiological stress associated with primary needs. There is a limited range of positive and negative signals (needs) that he must satisfy: hunger, pain, necessary needs, sleep. Each of these needs is absolutely vital and cannot be unsatisfied. Already in the 3rd-5th week of life, there is a need for social contact, but first with the person who makes it possible to survive. In the 3rd month, there is psychomotor animation and recognition of the mother or several persons most often in the child's field of vision. At the same time, the need for

emotional and social contacts increases (Serdyukovskaya G. N., 1985). If up to 2 years old motor development prevails, the subsequent period is characterized by fast cognitive development and improvement of speech.

Age 3 to 4 is one of the most important developmental periods that runs critically (the first age crisis). During this age period, the child becomes capricious, irritable, vulnerable, disobedient, overly fatigued, irritable, stubborn, protesting against the authority of adults, prone to psychogenic breakdowns. Internal discomfort, tension, high sensitivity to deprivation causing frustration (L.I.   Bozholevich,

1978) are also noted.

The importance of importance of the "I am system" (I am!) developing by this age - self-consciousness, self-esteem, desire of approval of the activity is emphasized. If the crisis is accompanied by these features in full, it already can be designated as a pre-neurotic condition (Desunis G., 1962). The first neurotic displays at this age are outwardly revealed by behavioral reactions (protest, refusal). Consequently, by age 3 or 4, the child has, though a small, but appreciable baggage of cognitive abilities, social experience, realized and unconscious needs and desires, has self-esteem, confidence (or uncertainty) about the future, and communication difficulties. The importance of this crisis is confirmed by the actual data, I.A. Shashkov (1983) has revealed, that during this period, the frequency of psychogenic disorders is three times higher than in subsequent years.

The second age crisis (5-7 years old) is characterized by great participation in its occurrence, along with biological factors, of social and psychological causes. At this age the foundation of the personality is formed. "To miss the years of childhood up to the age of 5.5 years in education means to destroy the foundation of the past" (Garbuzov V. I., 1980). With normal development by the age of 5-7 years, one's own internal position, psychological attitudes, a conscious understanding of one's place, role in the family or other micro-environment already arise. At the same time, the fragility of the nervous system, instability of mental equilibrium, readiness for pathological reaction is clearly shown in this age crisis. During the specified age period, the obligation to study, going to school becomes a need (Serdyukovskaya G. N., 1985). L.I. Bozholevich (1979) has revealed an important regularity - the child has more difficulties if he or she enters school later than 7 years old. During the second age crisis, the basis for occurrence of elementary neurotic reactions is a propensity to overfatigue and psychosomatic asthenization (sleep disorders, appetite, dizziness, loss of capacity for work, fatigue, propensity to fears, etc.). Upon entering school, social awareness is formed very quickly (attitude to others, to oneself, to learning, successes and failures, experiencing and overcoming them).

In his time, L. S. Vygotsky (1960) concluded that the main content of the child's mental development is a change in the functional structure of consciousness, the essence of which is that at each stage of ontogenesis there are different nervous connections, a different readiness for perception of new mental experiences. At the same time, at each following stage one or another mental process gradually begins to take on significance. Thus, in younger school age it is the development of thinking, which determines changes in all other mental processes.

The third age crisis is the longest (12-18 years old), most expressed, most difficult and of the greatest value for understanding of age-specific mental disorders. This crisis is called "transition" from childhood to adulthood, a period of tumultuous internal and external conflicts. Ch. Buhler (1931) divided the pubertal crisis into two phases - negative (12-14 years old) and positive (15-18 years old). The age boundaries of our study capture the "negative" phase of the pubertal crisis - the period of the greatest change in the child's personality in the transition to adolescence. The critical character of development during this period is explained by the incompleteness of formation of various organs and systems, and also the heightened reactivity resulting in extreme sensitivity to psychological traumas.

It should be noted that the pubertal crisis is not an amorphous static state, but a purely dynamic one; a process of adolescence that has stages and content. From the two main processes of maturation (physiological and psychological) form the main content of puberty. These processes are considered in close dynamic unity, although each of them retains a certain autonomy and unevenness in form, function, clinical and social significance. Physiological maturation includes, along with sexual metamorphosis, maturation of the central nervous system, formation of biological and physiological homeostasis, the system "hypothalamus - pituitary - adrenal cortex - sex glands", neurohumoral regulation.

Psychological development ends after puberty, and social development completes the maturation process as a whole. The psychological behavior of children at the stage of pubertal crisis is characterized by such features as anxiety, restlessness, impulsiveness, negativism, conflict, inconsistency of feelings, aggressiveness, tendency to sharp mood swings, melancholy (Buhler Ch, 1931; Gessel A., 1956) Sensitivity is characteristic - sensitivity to the assessment by others of the appearance, force, abilities, skills, in combination with excessive self-confidence, excessive criticism, disregard for the judgments of adults (Lichko, A. E., 1985; Gessel A., 1956), 1956), a combination of sensitivity with startling callousness, painful shyness with impudence, a craving for recognition with self-confidence, a rejection of the generally accepted rules with deification of casual idols, sensual fantasizing with dry wisdom (G. E. Sukhareva, 1974; A. E. Lichko, 1985); striving for philosophical generalizations, internal inconsistency of psyche, uncertainty of the level of pretensions, inclination to extreme positions (Levin K., 1960), egocentrism of adolescent thinking, propensity to theorizing (Piaget J., 1967), aspiration to release from child independence (Sparanger E., 1925), oppositional readiness, maximalism in estimations, intolerance of trusteeship, a variety of experiences (Lebedinskaya K. S., 1969, 1974).

2.1 Peculiarities of dysontogenesis of children with depressive symptoms

The doctrine of pathological ground in child psychiatry is closely connected with the concept of dysontogenesis (G. E. Sukhareva, 1959). Inclusion of dysontogenesis in the concept of "pathological ground" is specific for age-specific psychiatric pathology. As it is known, in "adult" psychiatry, this concept is rarely applied and only in relation to critical age periods (involutionary, senile).

Dysontogenesis is neither a syndrome nor a nosological form, but broadly refers to disorder, distortion of ontogenetic development as a result of various damaging factors - from genetic, early gross structural lesions of the brain and consequences of chronic mental diseases to functional delays and asynchrony of development of psychogenic or social origin. Essentially, we are talking about development with a mental defect or developmental abnormalities that manifest independently or are part of the structure of more complex clinical forms.

Dysontogenesis is a temporary or persistent violation of ontogenesis, the emergence of various kinds of pathological shifts in development at the organ, systemic, organismic and/or mental level. In the latter case, we speak about "mental dysontogenesis. It can be manifested by general or partial acceleration (acceleration of development), retardation (lag), asynchrony (a combination of acceleration of development of some functions, systems or components of the personality and delayed development of others), regression (revival of forms of reaction and functioning normal for an earlier age, but archaic for the child's present age). The term "dysontogenesis" (from Greek "dys" - deviation from the norm, "ontos" - being, and "genesis" - development) was first used by J. Schwalbe in 1927 to denote deviations of intrauterine formation of body structures from the normal course of development. In domestic defectology, these conditions are grouped into a group of developmental disorders (deviations).

In modern researches in the field of children's and teenage psychiatry (Isaev D.N., 1982; Gurieva V.A., Semke V.Y., Gindikin V.Y., 1994, etc.) and works of psychologists (Lebedinsky V.V., 1985) the position has appeared according to which understanding of age regularities of mental disorders and their diagnostics in children and teenagers is impossible without clear representation about correlations of clinic and mental development disorders - dysontogenesis. This position is also reflected in a number of international conciliatory documents ("The Beijing Rules", 1985; "The UN Convention on the Rights of the Child",

1989).

The age factor, according to V. V. Kovalev (1969), is one of the major, specific for mental diseases in children, and in borderline conditions, it has the leading pathogenetic role. Based on the biogenetic theory of a stage of individual development, V. V. Kovalev (1969, 1973) suggests that the pathogenetic basis of the mental phenomena predominating in various age periods of childhood is the mechanism of a shift of qualitatively different levels of pathological neuropsychological reactions to certain harms. The author allocates four basic age levels: 1) somatovetegetative (0-3 years); 2) psychomotor (4-10 years); 3) affective (7-12 years); 4) emotional-ideal (12-16 years).

Ontogenetically earlier is the somato-vegetative level, which is characterized by various variants of the neuropathic syndrome (increased general and vegetative excitability, propensity to disorders of digestion, feeding, sleep, neatness skills, etc.). In his recent works and presentations, V. V. Kovalev (1995) already defined this level as "somato-vegetative-instinctive", thereby emphasizing the urgency of the participation of innate mechanisms, types and behaviors in the neuropsychological reactions of young children. The uniform context of neuropathic and ethological mechanisms is traced in pathogenesis of psychosomatic disorders and pathological habitual actions in children and teenagers (Y. F. Antropov, Y. S. Shevchenko, 1999).

The author categorizes as the psychomotor reaction level the manifestations of the hyperdynamic syndrome, systemic neurotic and neurosis-like motor disorders - mutism, stuttering, tics, etc. According to the data of age physiology and morphology, at the age of approximately 6 to 12 years (the period of preschool and junior school age), the most intensive differentiation of functions of the motor analyzer occurs (A. A. Volokhov, 1965). By the age of 7, the nucleus of the cortical part of the motor analyzer acquires a cytoarchitectonic structure similar to that of this area of the adult cortex.

The affective level of neuropsychological reactions (V.V. Kovalev, 1973) is characterized by syndromes of psychopathologically differentiated fears, syndromes of the raised affective excitability, careers and vagrancy, which are overlapping the previous, but shifted to an older age. Nevertheless, despite the fact that these manifestations are also noted earlier (for example, fears), but it is at age 6-7 years that they acquire psychopathological delineation. It is also connected with the beginning of formation of self-consciousness by the end of the preschool period and with occurrence in the child of elementary ability to self-estimate subjective experiences (Elkonin D.B., 1960).

During the prepubertal and pubertal periods, an emotional-ideal level of reactivity is manifested, the basic feature of which is the occurrence of supernatural formations. If also in the case of normal

In the case of disturbed ontogenesis, characterized by general or partial retardation, acceleration, asynchrony or regression, various atypical combinations of "timely", "accelerated" and "archaic" can take place, and in this case, the age limits between the above levels of neuropsychological response are not rigid and naturally superimpose on each other.

mechanisms of adaptation, which determines the occurrence of dysontogenetic phenomena specific to childhood.

Initially, the term "dysontogenia" referred to deviations in the intrauterine development of the organism. Subsequently, the concept became more capacious, as different researchers began to link it to developmental disorders due to antenatal, perinatal and postnatal pathology. However, the term "dysontogenesis" itself became widely used only in the 1960s, especially in the study of adolescent psychiatry and psychology.

According to V.V. Kovalev (1995), mental dysontogenesis is expressed in various violations of the rate and timing of mental maturation as a whole and its individual components, as well as in violation of the ratio of components of a child's developing psyche. Manifestations of dysontogenesis of mental development are associated with the action of causal factors of biological and socio-psychological nature. The younger the child, the greater the role played as causes of mental disorders by biological factors (genetic, infectious, immunological, toxic, metabolic, etc.) that cause a relatively narrow range of forms of mental pathology (oligophrenia, mental retardation, residual-organic disorders, etc.). The causal role of socio-psychological factors increases with age, leading to an increase in the incidence of reactive states, depressions, neuroses, psychogenic pathological personality formation, and psychosomatic disorders.

Thus, the biological causes of developmental dysontogenesis include infections, injuries, intoxications, genetic anomalies, maternal toxicosis during pregnancy and other factors involved in the formation of the individual constitution. Depending on the time of their impact, intrauterine perinatal and postnatal dysontogenetic pathology is distinguished. Social and psychological causes of dysontogenesis include improper upbringing, psychotraumatic situations, acute and subacute mental trauma, emotional deprivation, etc. However, biological and social and psychological factors are closely connected. As I.V. Davydovsky and A.V. Snezhnevsky (1965) wrote, "... social factors... do not act directly on the person, but always refract in one way or another in the natural factors, in the biological basis of the person".

The following classification of dysontogenesis is the most popular in domestic child psychiatry: delayed, distorted and damaged development (G. E. Sukhareva, 1959). There is a classification in which there are direct correlations between the type of dysontogenesis and the nosological form: Irreversible underdevelopment (mental retardation) in oligophrenia, disharmonic development in psychopathies, regressive development in degenerative and ongoing organic diseases of the central nervous system; alternating type in asynchronous development, dissociated development in schizophrenia, sociogenic dysontogenesis in long-term, severe deprivation (Lebedinsky V. B., 1976; Stutte H., 1963).

A comparison of contemporary studies concerning the systematization of mental development disorders in childhood has nevertheless demonstrated the presence of significant discrepancies in the systematics and classifications of dysontogenesis. These discrepancies concern not only the designation and clinical interpretation of the main evolutionary phenomena (developmental delays; impaired, delayed, damaged, and distorted development), but also the key concept itself - "dysontogenesis. Diverse approaches to the problem cause difficulty in comparing the results of research and difficulties in their practical application.

The methodological approach to the diagnosis of mental disorders with various types and forms of dysontogenesis is currently being refined in the child-adolescent forensic psychiatric examination (E.V. Makushkin, 2002). E. Having made more exact clinical-psychopathological and forensic-psychiatric approaches, Makushkin (2001, 2002) allocated 8 forms of disorder. 1) Delayed development: a) abnormal behavioral deviations; b) asynchrony of maturation (retardation, acceleration); c) partial (sociogenic and somatogenic) infantilism; 2) disharmonious development; 3) delayed development; 4) distorted development; 5) defective development; 6) dissociative development; 7) impaired development; 8) pubertal dysontogenesis (disharmonious psychosexual maturation and development by dissociative type). Such grouping encompasses the main forms of dysontogenesis in adolescence, reflecting developmental disorders of the personality level, including forms of impaired development found in the structure of various nosological forms. This taxonomy does not include total underdevelopment (mental retardation, childhood autism, genetic forms of total dysontogenesis), highlighted as independent nosological forms with their own special clinic, specificity and age dynamics.

As a whole, sharing the opinion expressed by Ch. Wenar, P.K. Kerig (2000, 2004), that child and adolescent psychologists and psychiatrists need to recognize the connection between processes of normal and abnormal development, each of which has its own specifics. This requires identification at individual, personal, interpersonal and suprapersonal levels of the specific risk factors that predetermine the "trajectory of development" unique to each child. However, the systematics of the various forms of mental disorders caused by impaired evolutionary development itself still requires contemporary clinical and dynamic comprehension. For example, currently accepted international classifications of diseases (ICD-10, DSM-IV) are adequately criticized for failing to take into account the normal developmental dimension of age. Needless to say, it is difficult to qualify symptoms (criteria) of mental dysontogenesis at different stages of child development, since dysontogenesis is far from being a static condition and can have both positive and negative age dynamics. Similar difficulties can arise in the assessment of comorbid disorders within the framework of the child-adolescent psychopathology. In such complex cases, it becomes difficult to determine whether a multiple diagnosis is accurate, whether it results from a lack of clear distinctions between diagnostic categories, or whether it is due to different early manifestations of multiple forms of developmental psychopathology (Cantweell D. P., 1996; Wener Ch., 2004). Only clear clinical verification of changes in rate, massiveness, level and quality of development in many respects predetermines a correct diagnosis of the mental and behavioral disorders associated with dysontogenesis.

To estimate the features of dysontogenesis of children with depressive disorders the analysis of clinic and dynamics of quantitative components and disclosure of qualitative (structural) components of disturbed (distorted, disproportional, etc.) development was carried out, which allowed to allocate (structure) models at various nosological variants of the depressive syndrome. From a position of clinical and psychological method, the model of normal development is presented in statics (considered as an integral synchronized state), reflecting harmony of normal development. According to E. V. Makushkin (2002), in accordance with ontogenetic unity, the harmonious development of the child is represented by six basic interconnected structural components of the mental (psychological), psychophysiological and psychosocial functioning. Among these components are cognitive (gnostic, cognitive, intellectual), affective (emotional), volitional and behavioral (regulatory) - psychological components of mental development, as well as somatophysical (somatoendocrine) -

psychophysical and sexual - psychosexual components of development. Due to the fact that peculiarities of dysontogenesis of children with depressive syndrome were assessed in childhood, when the child's personality is in the initial (negative) stage of pubertal crisis, developmental ontogenesis was assessed according to five main components: conative, affective, volitional, physical and behavioral.

In our case, the physical component included somatophysical and psychosexual components of development. The clinico-dynamic model of normal mental development (Fig. 2) represents a harmonious structure consisting of five components mapped to each other in dynamics at three age intervals: the first crisis at 2-3 years old, the second at 5-7 years old, and the third at 12-14 years old (the negative stage of the pubertal crisis). The model is projected on two axes - time (t) and rate of development (T).

In the figure presented, the rate is a certain speed of movement of those or other structural components of development, and time is an indicator of the timeliness of maturation (structuring) of mental functions. Such a construction makes it possible to take into account the dynamics of normal maturation most completely, to analyze and subsequently compare variants of distorted development with the relative norm. It is necessary for clinical assessment of the child's condition, differential diagnostic evaluation, construction of a structural diagnosis, prevention of depressive disorders, decision-making on therapeutic and rehabilitative measures.

In studying the features of dysontogenesis of children with diagnosed schizophrenia depression, a careful study of the features of developmental ontogenesis of these children was conducted. At the same time, the main developmental parameters were considered

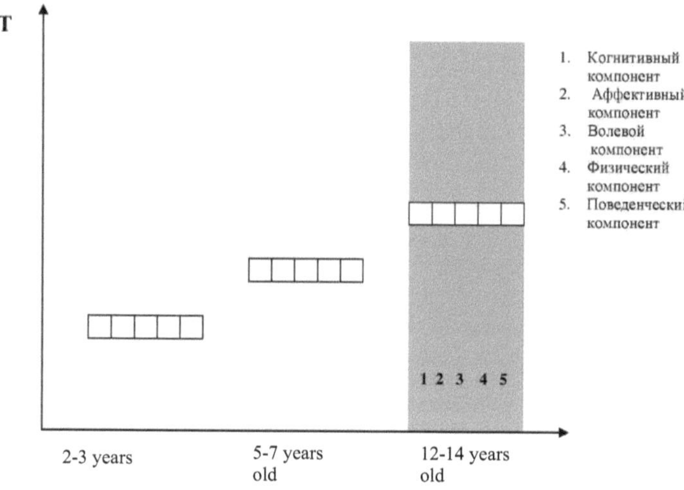

instinctive, emotional spheres, statistical functions, speech, play activity, formation of behavioral skills, relations with relatives. The clinical comparison revealed two **t**

Figure 2. Structural-dynamic model of normal development .

The first variant of dysontogenesis in depressed children with schizophrenia was characterized by "stratification," delayed formation and changes in the normal pace of development at all stages of developmental ontogenesis (Fig. 3). At the stage of the first crisis, there was a delayed formation of the structures of the cognitive and volitional components, dissociative formation of the emotional and behavioral components, and normal physical development.

Slow formation of the structure of the cognitive component was determined by some lagging behind peers in motor development and

• The structural-dynamic model of normal development proposed by E. V. Makushkin (2002). 69

70

The formation of phrasal speech, and mothers of children noted the emerging impression that children prefer to communicate with the help of gestures, fully understanding the speech addressed to them. Delayed formation of the volitional component was manifested by mild motor retardation, slowness of movements, decreased gesturing and delayed development of neatness skills. Children could not get used to using the potty for a long time, they later formed skills related to the development of fine motor skills (tying shoelaces, buttoning buttons, etc.).

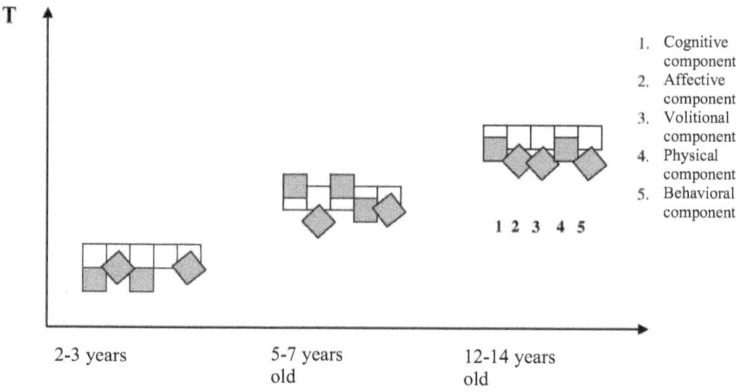

Fig. 3. The first structural-dynamic model
of dysontogenesis in depression in schizophrenia.

Changes in the emotional and behavioral components were manifested by low motor activity, reduced emotional reactions to recreational or distracting activities, they were characterized by some "seriousness" noted by their mothers. Such children were capricious and tearful throughout the day.

At the stage of the second crisis (5-7 years), acceleration of formation of the cognitive component with strengthening of the volitional, decrease and structural change in the affective and behavioral components with some lag in physical development was noted. Strengthening of formation of the cognitive component was manifested by early intellectual development of the child: children mastered reading and writing skills earlier, preferring literature recommended for older persons. Strengthening of the volitional component had a partial character: children showed uncharacteristic persistence in the affairs of interest and usual in others. The structural change of the behavioral and affective components was manifested by a change in the structure and form of socialization. Children were reluctant to communicate with surrounding children or completely refused to play together, their play activity was limited by the long-term fascination with one toy. At the stage of the third crisis (12-14 years old), there was a total asynchrony of development with a slight delay of the cognitive component related to the partiality of these children's interests, normal rates of physical development and pronounced asynchrony of the affective, volitional and behavioral components. Developmental disorders of the above components were manifested by difficulties in adapting to the children's group, difficulties in establishing social connections, refusal to communicate with peers, inactivity or unusual hobbies, increased tearfulness or constant readiness to cry, attacks of motor anxiety with screaming, crying, ridiculous threats and actions.

The second variant of dysontogenesis in depressed children with schizophrenia was characterized by a normal developmental rate in early childhood with an intensification of formation and a change in the normal developmental rate in the junior school and pre-adolescent years (Fig. 4).

At the stage of the first crisis, no disorders in the process of ontogenesis were detected: the formation of psychomotor functions took place within the physiologically normal periods for healthy children. During the first year of life, children formed emotional attachments to relatives and surrounding persons. From the second year, there was an expansion of contacts, including contacts with peers, and complex emotional reactions (joy, resentment) were formed.

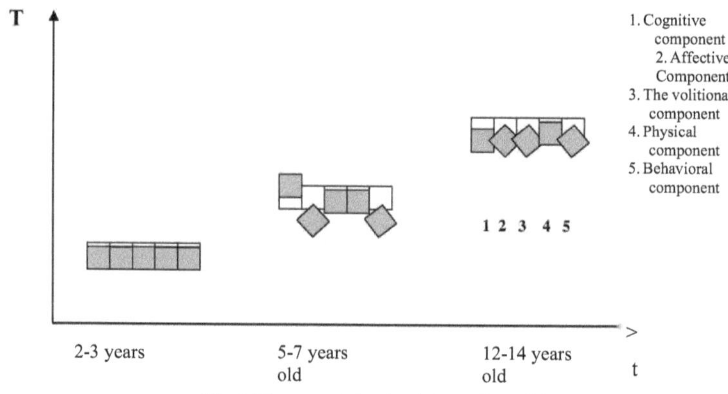

Fig. 4. The second structural-dynamic model
of dysontogenesis in depression on the background of
schizophrenia.

At the stage of the second crisis, acceleration of development of the cognitive component was noted: children were ahead of their peers in intellectual development. The volitional and physical components developed according to age norms. However, in the affective and behavioral spheres, there was a developmental asynchrony manifested in restriction of social contacts, changes in the development of higher emotional reactions, emotional detachment and lability of children. At the stage of the third crisis, a pronounced "stratification" and slowing down of the normal rate of development, expressed in asynchrony of affective, volitional and behavioral components of normal development, similar to the first variant of dysontogenesis of children with the depressive disorder on the background of schizophrenia, were shown.

Peculiarities of dysontogenesis of children with neurotic depressive disorders, we considered the main parameters of the development of instinctive, emotional sphere, statistical functions, speech, play activity, formation of behavioral skills, relationships with relatives. At the same time, no developmental disorders were noted in a part of the children. Dysontogenesis development was characterized by the absence of disruption of ontogenesis at the first stage   age crisis: the formation of psychomotor functions took place in physiologically normal times for healthy children (Fig. 5).

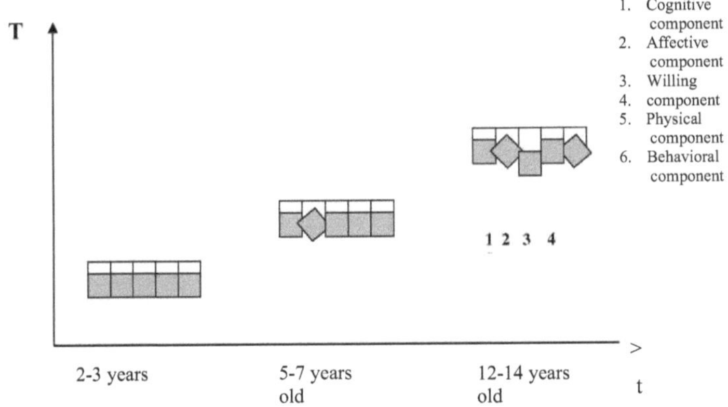

Fig. 5. Structural and dynamic model
dysontogenesis of children with neurotic depression.

At the second stage of the age crisis, formation of the cognitive, volitional, physical and behavioral components occurred in periods of the age norm. Asynchrony of development of the affective (emotional) component was noted, manifesting itself in excessive emotionality (friendliness, pity, some withdrawal). Children had difficulties at the beginning of socialization, at first they isolated themselves from socialization, refused to attend kindergarten, were capricious, cried; having gradually mastered, nevertheless kept their distance from the majority of children, preferring to communicate in the circle of relatives, warily reacting to strangers. At the stage of the third crisis, developmental dysontogenesis was manifested by a delayed formation of the volitional component and asynchrony of development of the affective and behavioral components of ontogenesis. Delayed formation of the volitional component was manifested in a decrease in the cognitive activity of the child (in the form of reduced mastering of subjects, a negative attitude to learning, refusal to attend school), weak willful activity in the school and home environment. Asynchrony of the affective and behavioral components was expressed in difficulty establishing social connections, conflictual relations with peers at school, motor disinhibition, tearfulness, fearfulness, mistrustfulness, withdrawal.

The features of dysontogenesis of children with depressive mood disorders on the background of mental retardation were determined by underdevelopment of the main components of normal ontogenesis, but the presence of depressive symptomatology determined additional asynchronization of separate components. Studying the features of dysontogenesis of these children, two basic forms of impaired development were revealed.

The first variant of dysontogenesis in children with a depressive syndrome against the background of mental retardation was characterized by a slower rate of formation of all components of child development with changes in individual components (Fig. 6).

The stage of the first age crisis in children with mental retardation was characterized by retardation of all components of normal developmental ontogenesis, irreversible underdevelopment in the formation of static and locomotor functions, understanding and reproduction of speech, intellect and personality of the child (Isaev D. N., 1982; Kovalev V. V., 1983; Lebedinsky V. V., 1985; Lutz J., 1968).

At the stage of the second age crisis, there was a stratification of the cognitive, affective, volitional and physical components with a predominant delay of intellectual development and a decrease in volitional activity of the child. At the same time, the lag in affective and physical development was less pronounced. During the first to second year of life, children formed emotional attachments to relatives and surrounding persons. In the third year of life, complex emotional reactions (joy, resentment) were formed. Asynchrony of the behavioral component was manifested in delayed expansion of contacts with peers, children preferred spend time among relatives, have had difficulty adapting to the children's team, were withdrawn, quiet, inconspicuous, resentful and fearful.

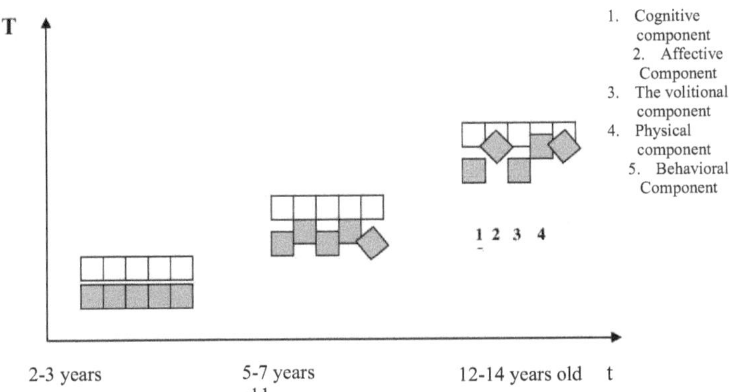

Fig. 6. The first structural-dynamic model of dysontogenesis of children
with a depressive syndrome on the background of mental retardation.

The third stage of development was characterized by a pronounced "stratification" of the affective and behavioral components with a characteristic delay of cognitive and volitional activity and slight physical underdevelopment. Asynchrony of affective and behavioral components was manifested by decreased adaptive capacities in the children's environment, children did not communicate with peers, limited social contacts, were irritable, conflictual, withdrawn, whiny, remained inactive in the home; time was mostly spent watching children's television programs.

The second variant of dysontogenesis of children with a depressive syndrome on the background of mental retardation and was characterized not only by a slower rate of formation of all components of child development, but also by changes in individual components from the beginning of the first age crisis (Fig. 7).

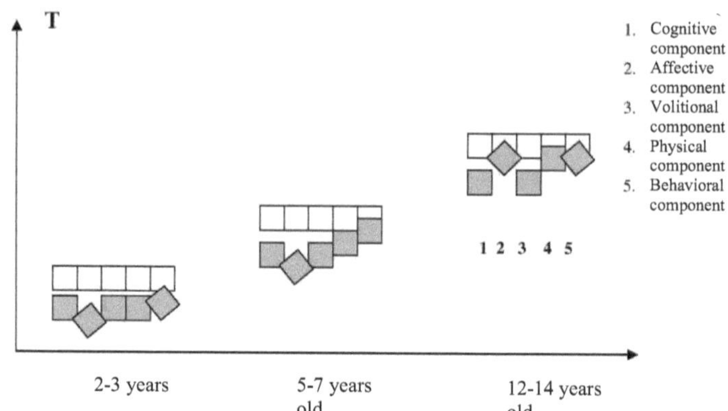

Fig. 7. The second structural-dynamic model of dysontogenesis of children with a depressive syndrome on the background of mental retardation.

In this variant of dysontogenesis, the first stage of the age crisis was characterized by retardation of all components of normal development, characteristic of all children with mental retardation and asynchrony of the affective component, manifested by irritability, capriciousness, tearfulness, lethargy. These children's sleep was characterized by restlessness; they had trouble falling asleep, often woke up at night and were calmed down only in their mother's arms. An inversion of daily rhythm was observed in some children. The formation of complex emotional reactions occurred much later than in children in the first group. At the stage of the second age crisis, marked asynchrony in the development of all components (cognitive, affective, volitional, physical and behavioral) was observed. Thus, the development of the cognitive and volitional components corresponded to the basic diagnosis of mental retardation. Physical underdevelopment was insignificant. The behavioral component was sufficiently developed and was characterized by a rather high social activity of the child (children willingly visited preschool institutions, communicated with other children, participated in public events). Against this background, uneven development of the emotional

Children were fearful, capricious, and whiny. The third age crisis proceeded similarly to the first variant of a course of dysontogenesis of children with the depressive syndrome on a background of mental retardation.

The features of dysontogenesis in children with organic depressive disorders were also considered by us in parallel with the study of the main parameters of the development of the instinctive, emotional spheres, statistical functions, speech, play activities, formation of behavioral skills, relationships with relatives. Comparing the formation of the main components of normally ongoing ontogenesis, we identified two forms of dysontogenesis.

The first variant of dysontogenesis was characterized by a delayed formation of the cognitive and volitional components with asynchrony of development of the affective, volitional and behavioral components at all stages of personality development (Fig. 8).

The stage of the first age crisis proceeded with a slight delay in the formation of the cognitive and volitional components of ontogenesis, and a delay in the formation of motor-static functions and the formation of speech skills was detected. Asynchrony and delay of the behavioral component in the form of excessive tearfulness, caprice, lethargy and low activity was characteristic of young children, with reduced ability to purposeful actions, retardation and general motor imperfection, which was reflected in play activity, in mastering self-care skills and intellectual skills. The change of the affective component of development was manifested by neurosis-like symptomatology with sleep and appetite disorders.

This variant of dysontogenesis due to early organic brain damage was reflected by the syndrome of "organic neuropathy" (A.E. Lichko, 1979; D.N. Isaev, 1984) or a neuropath-like version of a psycho-organic syndrome (V.V. Kovalev, 1979).

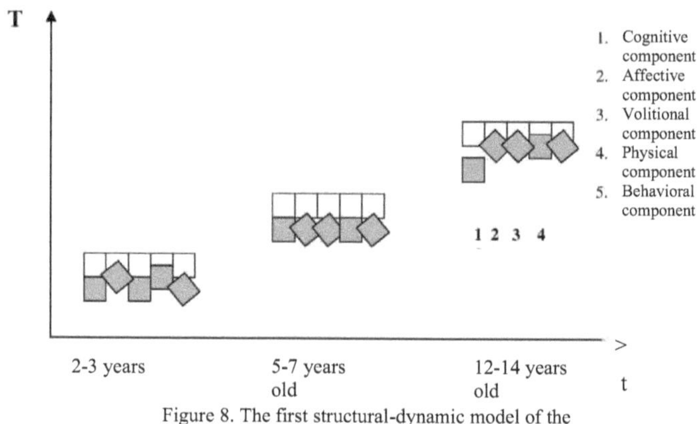

Figure 8. The first structural-dynamic model of the
development of children
with affective depressive disorder.

At the second stage there was a retardation of all components of ontogenesis with a change in the normal course of the affective, volitional and behavioral components, manifested in a decrease in the child's social activity, adaptive abilities, low sociality, fearfulness. The stage of the third age crisis was characterized by a pronounced decrease in the cognitive component, manifesting itself in difficulty to master the school program with preservation of asynchrony of the affective, volitional and behavioral components, acquiring more developed forms, with strengthening of irritability, negativity, disorganization, emotional lability, etc., typical for this age.

The second variant of dysontogenesis was characterized by relatively harmonious development at the stage of the first crisis with the appearance of asynchrony of the affective and behavioral components at the stage of the second and a decrease in the cognitive and volitional components at the stage of the third age crisis (Fig. 9).

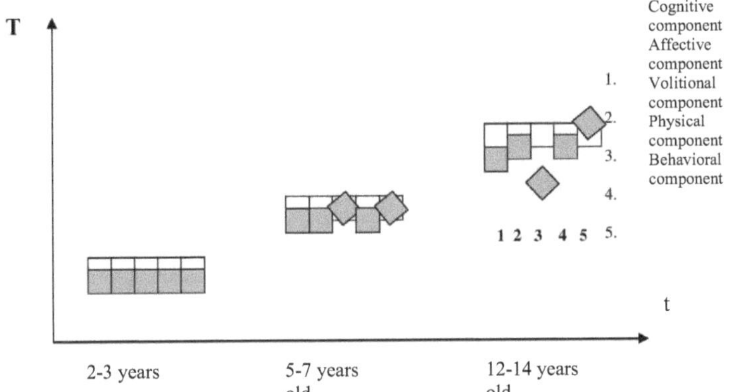

Figure 9. The second structural-dynamic model of dysontogenesis of children with affective depressive disorder.

At the stage of the first age crisis, no deviations were found in the normal course of the coontogenesis; the formation of all the main components took place in physiologically normal terms, without changes in the structure. The second crisis was characterized by rather normal development of the cognitive, affective and physical components, with the appearance of asynchrony of development of the volitional and behavioral components. Children were irritable, conflictive, aggressive in relation to relatives and surrounding children, selfish, motor-disordered, and also displayed aspiration to take the lead and rule. At the stage of the third crisis, a pronounced structural change of components of development with retardation of the cognitive and volitional components, asynchrony of the volitional and behavioral components, acceleration of the rate of development of the behavioral component, which was expressed in a decrease in the child's intellectual development with a marked decrease and change of volitional activity (difficulties in mastering the school program with refusal to attend educational institutions and a desire to join teenage asocial groups) was observed. Simultaneously, there was an amplification of development of socialization of the child with change of the behavioral patterns peculiar to adolescence.

Thus, studying the developmental ontogenesis of children with the depressive syndrome, it was found that the disorder of normal developmental ontogenesis occurred in almost all nosological groups of children with depressive disorders, but the nosological affiliation determined different forms of the course of dysontogenetic conditions. However, the types of dysontogenesis were not static in their characteristics, they were distinguished by a certain clinical dynamics (with pathoplastic and multidimensional syndrome forms), reflecting the specifics of disturbed age-related development.

2.2 Social development of children with depressive symptoms

The process of social development in ontogenesis has a multistage character and is carried out throughout life in different directions. It is accepted to distinguish several periods of ontogenesis: 1) period newbornness; 2) infancy; 3) the preschool period; 4) the preschool period; 5) the school period; 6) the adulthood period; 7) old age. There is another widespread periodization of development developed by D. Elkonin (1989) - infancy (the leading kind of activity is direct emotional dialogue); early childhood (object-manipulative actions); preschool childhood (role-play); younger school childhood (educational activity); adolescence (intimate-personal dialogue); youth (educational-professional activity). The phases of the life course imprint on the age stages of ontogenesis to such an extent that at present some age stages are designated exactly as phases of the life course: preschool, preschool, childhood, school.

Social maturation has its own course, its own character, its own levels of development, integrating all other achievements of ontogenesis, since social maturity most fully expresses the maturity of a personality. Disclosure of the process of personality development implies a thorough analysis of its origins, conditions, factors determining its formation, consideration of its genesis, peculiarities of movement and functioning. In this case it is necessary to focus not only on what is actually available, but also on what should be formed in the personality (Kovalev A. G., 1965; V. V. Davydov, 1972; D. I. Feldstein, 1976, 1982; A. A. Bodalev, 1982).

Meanwhile, it is activity that serves as a constant substrate of human development as a person. Only by mastering the system of activity set by society in the process of upbringing, the child develops as a person, is formed as a transformer of society and himself. In this connection, it is important, first, to trace the nature of personality development through the development of activity; and second, to consider stages of personality formation as a special form of development of the generic, social essence of man.

Guided by the activity-based approach to the formation of a person as a personality established in psychology, we study the process of a child's mastering new social positions and appropriation of human essence as a result of movement and development of activity, bearing in mind two points. On the one hand, in activity, its subject-object and subject-subject lines, which are forms of realization of a person's social essence, the child's development occurs as a disclosure of his or her inner possibilities. On the other hand, we are faced with a specially set activity, which is a condition of human development as a personality. Organized by society (external), activity creates the situation in which the child's attitudes, needs, consciousness and self-consciousness (internal activity) are formed. Therefore, when studying personality development in ontogenesis, we focus our attention on the search for opportunities to build a system of externally set activity that provides real restructuring of the child's internal activity and formation of a motive for this activity. Thus, as R. Lewontin (1993): "The correct understanding of the origins of human "nature" and the diversity of people is determined by understanding two fundamental features of the organism: first, each organism is a subject of constant development throughout its life; second, the developing organism is under the joint influence of interacting genes and environment at any given time".

Society always sets the standard for the individual, whose development process is aimed at mastering the social world, its objects and relations, historically developed forms and ways of dealing with nature and norms of human relationships, that is, at the appropriation of the social human essence by the growing person. Hence, ontogenesis acts as a form of social development of man, his formation as a being of the social, with different age stages characterized by differences in self-knowledge, self-actualization, creative activity, social maturity. Such approach to consideration of ontogenetic development through the prism of social movement provides search of new reserves of personal formation and possibilities of optimization of educational influence taking into account periods of special openness of the developing person to social influences.

Based on the cardinal provisions, we assume that in the process of ontogenesis, a growing person masters social experience, appropriates it, makes it his property, i.e. socialization takes place. At the same time, man acquires more and more independence, relative autonomy, i.e. there is his individualization. In fact, these are inextricably interrelated components of a single process of personal development, a certain level of which generates self-determination, self-government of the individual, consciously organizing his own life, and, therefore, determining to some extent his own development. But a child becomes a personality, a subject, a bearer of socio-human activity only as a result of this activity performed first with the help of adults, and then independently. The child is not born a person, but develops as a person in the course of the development of activity and goes beyond the given activity. Although personality in general is a result of ontogenetic development, manifesting itself at its certain stages, but as a quality that expresses the social essence of man, personality begins to be formed from birth.

Without setting out to consider the entire complex, multidimensional problem of personality, understanding that in its development as a "supersensible" (Leontiev A. N.., 1983, vol. I, p. 385) as a social individual, intertwine in its integral totality mental, psychophysiological, moral-volitional, needs-motivational and other components, we believe it necessary in this work to highlight the core, structure-forming moments that express the degree of development of the child's socialization as a personality in conventional social institutions (family, preschool institutions, school).

At the early stages of a child's development (up to the age of 3), the family as the closest social object of environment, in particular the structure and wholesomeness of the family, the forms of upbringing adopted in this social unit, the psychological climate, the educational level of parents, is of the greatest importance in the formation of socialization. At further developmental stages (3-7 years), the factor of the child's inclusion in the social environment - the environment of peers - acquires significance: attendance of preschool institutions, features of adaptation in the children's environment (play activity, formation of friendly, role patterns of behavior). At the next stage of development (7 years and older), due to the child's rapid intellectual development, there is a tangible need to accumulate not only social, but also intellectual experience, i.e. to educate the child in school. In the given age period compulsory education, going to school becomes a need (Serdyukovskaya G. N., 1985). It is expedient to study social development of children with a depressive syndrome in the following basic directions.

<u>Family environment</u>: 1) family structure (presence of both parents, grandparents; adoptive parents; social care authorities); 2) psychological climate in the family (presence of emotional attachment to the child, relations between relatives); 3) presence of pathological forms of upbringing; 4) educational and general cultural level of the family.

<u>Preschool institutions</u>: 5) attendance at preschool; 6) age of starting to attend preschool; 7) adaptation of the child to preschool (play activities, presence of friendly relationships with peers, preferred social circle).

<u>School</u>: 8) age of beginning school attendance; 9) adequacy of the educational program to the intellectual development of the child; 10) ability to master the school program; 11) adaptation of the child in the peer environment.

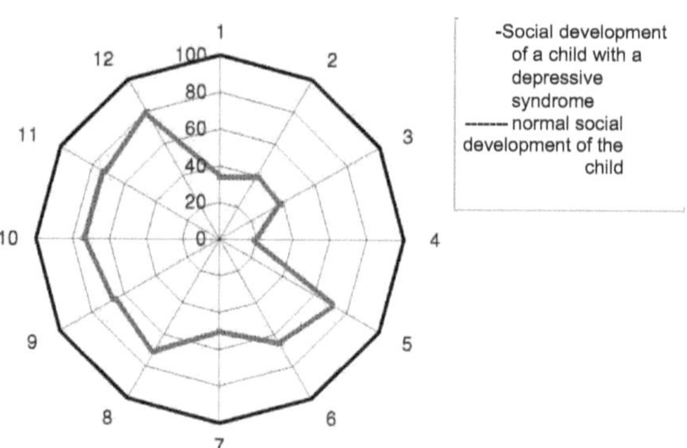

Figure 10. Social development of a child with depressive disorders.

Note to Fig. 10, 11, 12, 13, 14: 1 - Absence of pathological types of parenting in the family, 2 - Absence of violations of emotional relations between parents, 3 - Absence of violations of the family structure, 4 - Absence of changes in the psychological climate in the family, 5 - High general cultural and educational levels of parents, 6 - Attending preschool, 7 - Starting to attend preschool at a normal age (3 years), 8 - No violations of child adaptation in preschool, 9 - Age at starting school at 7, 10 - Educational program matched the intellectual development of the child, 11 - No adaptation violations

Studying features of social development of children with depressive disorders (DR), it has been established that at all stages of development there were expressed disorders of socialization (Fig. 10).

In the early stages of development, there was a change in the microclimate, emotional relationships and family structure. Only a small fraction of children were raised in full families by full parents, with opportunities to expand emotional attachment and form the basic structural and gender bases of interaction.

The normal psychological climate in the families was observed only in 18.8% of those surveyed, in the remaining cases (81.2%) relations between the parents were assessed as conditionally favorable, conflictual or emotionally rejected. Pathological forms of upbringing were identified in 66.3% of families with children with depressive disorders. At the same time, violation of emotional contact with a child in the form of emotional rejection was noted in 60.8% of those surveyed, imbalance of emotional attachment between several children or complete rejection of a child by parents with his or her transfer to adoptive parents or orphanages in 14.1%. Socialization in children with PD at the stage of becoming socially active and determining their place in social institutions and peer groups was also impaired. Thus, 36.4% of children did not attend preschool educational institutions, and 50.0% of children started attending kindergartens when they were younger than 2 years old or older than 5 years old. Among the children who attended preschool educational institutions, 29.3% had difficulties in communicating with their peers, which was expressed in impaired play activities and isolation from the social environment.

At the third stage of development (the school-age period), there were still disorders: 21.9% of children began attending school when they were older than 8 years old; 26.3% had an educational program that did not match their intellectual development (in particular, children with mental retardation or intellectual disabilities were taught in a general education school); 20.5% of children had significant problems in mastering program material; 26.9% had problems adjusting to school (they had difficulties forming friendships, determining peers). Making a comparison at different age stages, it was determined that the child's socialization was disturbed mostly at the early age stages in the immediate family environment and at the stage of acquiring the first social experience (preschool).

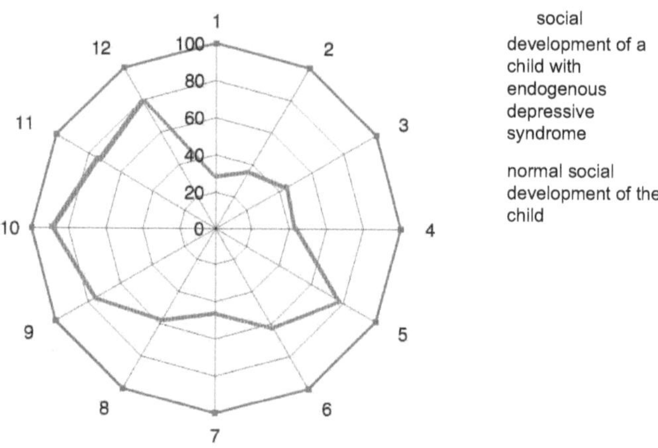

Fig. 11. Social development of a child with a
depressive syndrome against the background of
schizophrenia.

Considering the social development of depressed children with schizophrenia (Fig. 11), it was revealed that in children from this group the disorders of normal development occur to a greater extent at the stage of early personality development (family environment). 56.3% of the children were brought up in single-parent families or in families with an altered structure (guardians, adoptive parents). In 57.3% of the families there was a violation of the psychological climate in the family, the parents' relationship was characterized by dysfunctional, emotional rejection (there were frequent quarrels and scandals in the family). The educational level of the parents was rather high - 77.3% of the parents had a specialized secondary or higher education, also in this group parents often had one (22.7%) or several higher educations (15.2%).

Children in this group attended preschool in most cases (61.9%), but their social activity was altered and 42.1% of children had pronounced adaptation disorders (they played independently in kindergarten, did not participate in collective games, did not establish friendly contacts with peers; in addition, due to their peculiar behavior, such children were often rejected by their peer group and experienced constant insults). In general, children started attending school on time, but 24.9% of those surveyed in this group started attending school at age 6 due to their active intellectual development. 10.9% of children had no interest in learning because they were intellectually ahead of their peers, which affected these children's adaptation to school. 26.5% had difficulties in social communication, similar to those in preschool (still rejected from the social environment, experiencing persecution from their peers).

Thus, the SR of children with depressive disorder on the background of schizophrenia was characterized by disharmonious formation at the stage of family environment (all constituent elements), the beginning of disorders from the period of attending preschool institutions (when establishing contacts with peers) with gradual leveling off toward normalization of socialization during school age.

Studying the features of social development of children with organic depressive disorders (Fig. 12), already at the stages of early development were found pronounced changes in the psychological climate in the family, only in 24.5% of the children surveyed had family relationships of the emotional attachment character, in 49.1% of children upbringing had a relatively harmonious character.

An altered family structure occurred in 36.3% of those surveyed, 28.1% of the children were being raised by a single parent (mothers who divorced the children's fathers), as a result of which 41.8% of them had pronounced emotional disorders between the parents (quarrels, scandals, conflicts in the presence of children). These disturbed relations had a clear impact on the early socialization of the children. Most of the children (70.1%) attended kindergartens, but 45.4%

of the children were forced to attend kindergartens when they were younger than 3 years old due to a variety of problems, and 45.4% had difficulty adjusting (either avoiding their peers or exhibiting aggressive tendencies toward the children around them).

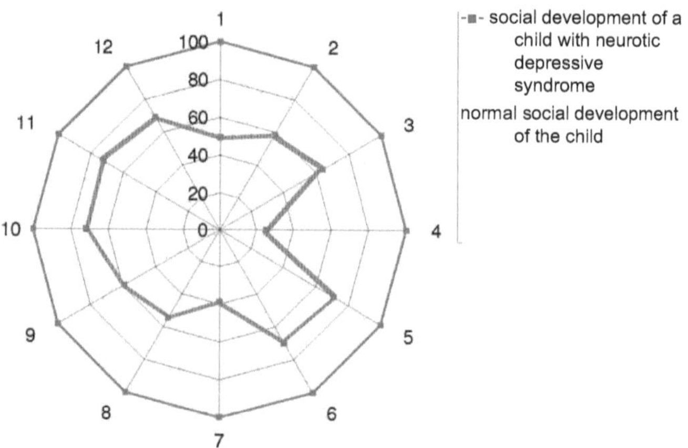

Figure 12. Social development of a child with an organic depressive syndrome.

They started school somewhat later than the age corresponding to normal SR, 23.6% were older than 8 years of age. Only a small proportion of children in this group had difficulty learning the school curriculum (28.1%) and adapting to the school environment (28.1%); in addition, children aspired to take leadership positions, and failures in this often led to conflicting relationships with peers.

Thus, the following components of social development were most typical for children with organic depressive disorders: pathological types of upbringing in the family, violation of the psychological family climate, early age of onset

Attendance at preschools, conflictual relations with peers at school age.

Peculiarities of social development of children with depressive mood disorders on the background of mental retardation (Fig. 13) were characterized by retardation of all moments of normal ontogenesis, at all stages of child development. At the age of up to 3 years, children were raised in families where parents had low cultural and educational levels.

Thus, only 50.0% of the parents had a high school education, and 50.0% of the children were raised in families with a modified structure. The relatively harmonious type of upbringing was detected only in 31.3% of the families, and the prevailing type among the forms of improper upbringing was neglect (27.1%). A large number of violations were noted at the stage of attendance of preschool institutions.

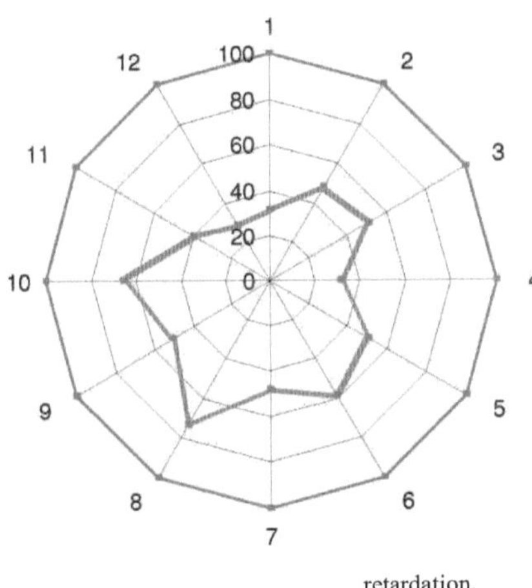

Fig. 13. Social development of a child with a depressive syndrome against a background of mental

Only 58.3% of the children attended kindergarten, of whom 52.1% were older than 5 years of age, but among them only 28.1% had difficulties in social adaptation in the community, associated with general intellectual underdevelopment.

At the stage of schooling, 49.8% of children began attending school when they were older than 8 years old. In 34.4% the educational program did not correspond to their intellectual development (children with mental retardation studied according to the program of a general education school). Most of the children (60.4%) had difficulties in mastering the school program and adapting to their peers (71.8%).

Thus, in the group of children with depressive disorders on the background of mental retardation, there was a violation of social development, namely

pronounced underdevelopment at all stages of social ontogenesis with predominant retardation during school age.

Impairment of social development in children with neurotic depressive disorder (Fig. 14) began already at the stage of early socialization of the child (up to the age of 3 years) and was connected with the nearest family environment.

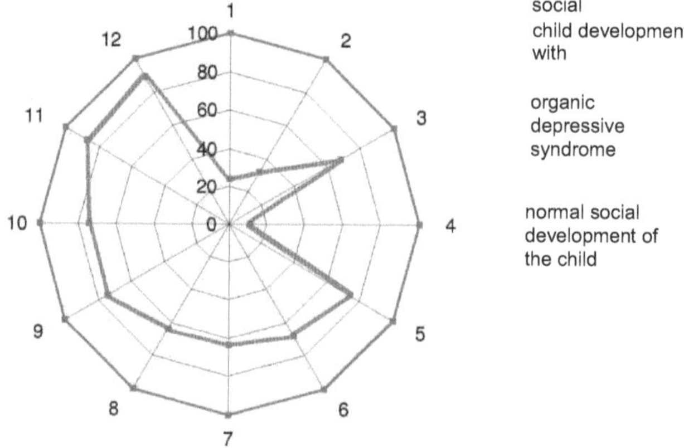

Fig. 14. Social development of a child with a
neurotic depressive syndrome.

In the families of these children there were significant changes in the psychological climate (89.1%), violation of emotional ties between the parents - 68.9% (frequent quarrels between the parents, physical methods of punishment for these children), pathological forms of upbringing (76.5%), in among which the "family idol" type of upbringing prevailed - 23.5%. However, as the child grew up, there was a smooth alignment of the social activity of the child with its maximum approximation to normal at the stage of school age.

Thus, among children with neurotic depressive disorders, the structure of social development disorders is characterized by a significant delay in the early stages of ontogenesis due to changes in the psychological climate of the family and the presence of pathological forms of upbringing with gradual compensation during school age.

The identified SR delays in children with DR make it necessary to determine the social age of the child with the identified depressive disorder. Assessment of influence of the revealed depressive syndrome on socialization of the child was carried out with use of the Doll Social Competence Scale (VSMS) (Doll E. A., 1953) modified by V. I. Gordeev, Yu. S. Aleksandrovsky (2001), the essence of which is to simplify the procedure of calculation of the received result.

Social competence can be defined as a child's ability to ensure personal independence and social responsibility. This competence can be measured in age dynamics on the basis of the individual's genetically determined maturation, which is diagnosed by age-appropriate psychosocial tests - paragraphs. Individual status in the sphere of social competence can be rearranged numerically and descriptively and characterized in relation to the norms of psychosocial maturity established in a given place and time. The use of this scale makes it possible to assess the subject's social age (SA - social age), and on the basis of this to determine the social quotient (SQ - social quotient) of the relationship between social age and chronological age. Each paragraph of the scale is labeled with age and category, which are subscales. SHG (self help general), general self-care; SHE (selfhelp eating), self-care in eating; SHD (selfhelp dressing), self-care in dressing; SD (self-direction), independence; O (occupation), employment; C (communication), communication; L (locomotion), meaningful, purposeful movement; S (socialization), socialization. Examining the social age of children with depressive symptomatology, a lag in social maturation with a predominant decrease in the child's developmental process was revealed (Fig. 15).

Children with depressive disorders on the background of schizophrenia during the age period of 8-9 years were characterized by being ahead of the chronological age due to independence, employment, and communication.

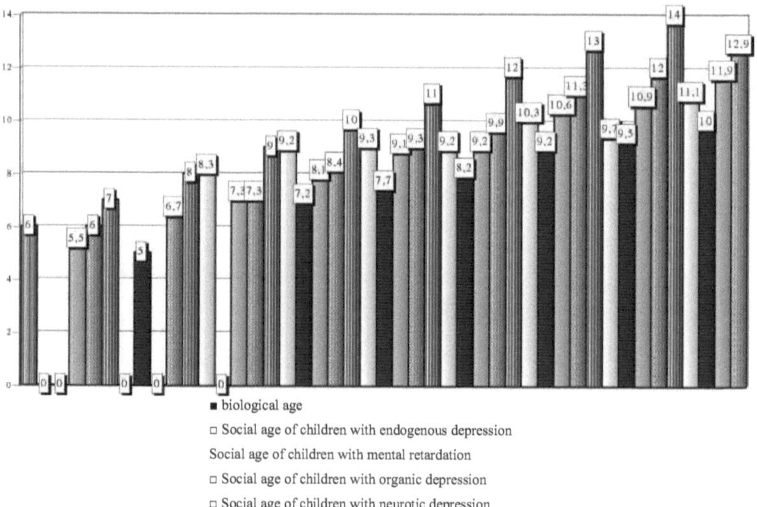

Figure 15. Correlation of biological and social age
in children with depressive disorders.

Table 1

Age-specific social quotient of children with identified depressive symptoms

Social ratio	Chronological age, years								
	6	7	8	9	10	11	12	13	14
Children with depression in schizophrenia	0	0	1,04	1,02	0,93	0,83	0,85	0,74	0,79
Children with depression on the background of mental retardation	0	0,71	0	0,8	0,77	0,74	0,76	0,73	0,71
Children with organic depression	0,91	0	0,91	0,9	0,91	0,83	0,88	0,83	0,85
Children with neurotic depression	1	0,95	0,91	0,93	0,93	0,9	0,94	0,92	0,92

Thus, at this age stage, the social coefficient was 1.04 and 1.02 points, reaching 104 and 102% of the norm of social maturity. From the age of 10 there was a smooth decrease in the child's socialization (0.93; 0.83; 0.85; 0.74; 0.79) due to a decrease in general self-care, independence, communication, and locomotion skills. Consequently, for the 10-year-old child population, social maturity was 93%, age 11 was 83.0%, age 12 was 85.0%, age 13 was 74.0%, and age 14 was 79.0% (Table 1).

For children with depressive disorders on the background of mental retardation, there was a significant delay in SR at all age stages with a predominant decrease in the age of starting school (age 7 - 0.71) and as they got older (0.8; 0.77; 0.74;, 0.76; 0.73; 0.71). This decrease was associated with a decrease in the following socialization categories: general self-care, employment, communication, independence, socialization. Consequently, at age 7 and 14, a child's socialization was 71.0% of the social maturity norm. For children aged 9 years old, social maturity was 80.0%, 10 years old was 77.0%, 11 years old was 74.0%, 12 years old was 76.0%, and 13 years old was 73.0%.

Children with organic depressions had a slight lag in social age from chronological age up to 10 years (0.91) mainly due to a decrease in locomotion skills, independence, accounting for 91.0% of social maturity. From age 11 there was a sharp decrease in the child's social competence (0.83; 0.88; 0.83; 0.85) due to impaired categories of independence, employment, and communication. Social maturity was 83.0% for 11-year-olds, 88.0% for 12-year-olds, 83.0% for 13-year-olds, and 85.0% for 14-year-olds.

Children with neurotic depression had a slight decrease in social age versus chronological age (0.95; 0.91; 0.93; 0.93; 0.90; 0.94; 0.92; 0.92) due to decreased socialization and communication of children. Thus, the social maturity of these children was 100.0% at age 6, 95.0% at age 7, 91.0% at age 8, 93.0% at age 9, 93.0% at age 10, 90.0% at age 11, 94.0% at age 12, 92.0% at age 13, and 92.0% at age 14.

Thus, the social development of children with depressive disorder on the background of schizophrenia was characterized by disharmonious formation at the stage of family environment and the stage of early socialization associated with attendance of preschool institutions with a gradual alignment toward normalization during school age. For children with an organic depressive syndrome, disharmony of socialization at an early age due to pathological types of parenting in the family and disorders of the psychological family climate were most typical, with this trend persisting while attending preschool and school. For children with depressive disorders on a background of mental retardation, a pronounced underdevelopment at all stages of social ontogenesis with predominant retardation during school age was typical. In children with neurotic depressive disorders in the structure of disorders of social ontogenesis of development, a significant retardation at the early stages of ontogenesis with gradual compensation during school age prevailed.

Comparing social coefficients of children depending on the nosological affiliation of the depressive disorder   , we found that the lowest rates of social maturity were characteristic of children with depressive disorders with mental retardation due to impaired general self-care, employment, communication, independence, socialization   skills. In children with depressive disorders with schizophrenia in the early school age there was even some advance of social age at 8-9 years with a sharp decrease later due to impairment of general self-care, independence, communication and locomotion skills. In children with organic depressive disorders, a significant decrease in social competence occurred from the age of 11 years, mainly due to impairment of independence, employment, and communication. To a lesser extent, impairment of social competence was characteristic of children with neurotic depressive disorders and was caused by deviations in the spheres of socialization and communication.

CHAPTER III.
CLINICAL AND DYNAMIC FEATURES OF THE COURSE OF DEPRESSIVE
MOOD DISORDERS IN CHILDREN

Most psychiatrists believe that depressive disorders are a frequent component of many mental illnesses, influencing their essence and structure, with early identification of the nosological identity of the disorder necessary to determine prognosis and therapeutic approaches (Tiganov A. S. et al., 1986; Iovchuk N. M., 1999; Mosolov S. N., 1995; Panteleeva G. P., 1999). There are various syndromological systematizations of depressive disorders in children, which have no uniform grouping criteria and separately do not reflect a variety of phenomenological variants of depression. Most often, DPs were divided according to the predominant affect in the clinical picture. H. Kielholz (1980) divided depression into four basic forms: with melancholy and depression, with anxiety and agitation, apathetic forms and larvic conditions with neurovegetative and psychosomatic symptoms. M. Kovacs (1984) singles out "major depression", dysthymia and adaptation disorder with depression in schoolchildren.

H. Remschmidt (1973) classified circular depression in terms of phenomenological features, distinguishing between inhibited, agitated, hypochondriacal, and phobic variants. V.M. Bashina et al. (1999) have considered MD within the framework of 8 most frequent types in children: adynamic, asthenic, anxious, dreary, melancholic, psychopathoid, dysphoric, somatized, with accession of a group of depressive states, one of which leading symptoms was anorectic behavior. N. M. Iovchuk, A. A. Severny's (1999) division into types of depression in children is based on the definition of the leading disorder that dominates over other depressive symptomatology and does not disappear during periods of its temporary weakening.

Taking into account the features of the clinical picture, 14 variants of depression in childhood have been described in general: simple, wistful, anxious, fearful, tearful, dysphoric, stuporous, with psychopathic-like disorders, adynamic, asthenic-like, stupid, anesthetic and somatized, and "adolescent asthenic insolence".

F. Antropov (2001) allocated the following typological variants of neurotic depression on the basis of the clinico-psychopathological features, on the basis of the accompanying affective displays of hypothymia: anxious, asthenic, asthenic-trevotic, anxious-dreary. V. I. Posokhova (1982), E. S. Natalevich et al. (1982) allocate asthenic, anxious, dysphoric, hysterical and hypochondriac among the variety of clinical variants of reactive depression existing in psychiatric practice. V. A. Gurieva, V. J. Semke, V. Ya. Gindikin (1994) propose the following typology of depression: Asthenodepressive state ("anxious" and "sluggish" variants); typical melancholic depression; depression with motor retardation; dysphoric depression; somatized or masked depression ("hyperkinetic" and "hypokinetic" variants, hypochondriac, asthenoaptic, delinquent equivalents); associatively accelerated depression. In evaluating this classification, it is easy to see that it includes both typical depression (indeed, little different from adult depression) and atypical depression. Such a differentiated approach to the phenomenology of depression taking into account the rate of individual physical and mental development of the teenager, according to M. G. Usov (1996), seems to be flexible enough and aimed to develop more accurate diagnostic criteria.

There are other approaches to the study of depression with behavioral disorders. N. M. Iovchuk (1989) divided psychopathic-like depressions by the type of a leading affect into two variants of depressive states: dysphoric depression and Unlust-depression. The main differences of these two groups were the presence of accessory symptoms in Unlust-depression, ideas of unjust treatment, with aggression being limited to the family circle, suicidal behavior, which could be explained by the endogenous process, since Unlust-depression was observed predominantly in the schizophrenic structure. A. E. Lichko (1979) described in detail three depressive equivalents: delinquent, hypochondriacal and asthenoapathic. O. D. Sosiukalo et al. (1983), V. V. Kovalev (1985) consider the term "delinquent equivalent of depression" inappropriate and propose to call it "a psychopath-like version of depression".

Using the traditional classification of P. Kielholz (1972), which is based on the nosological principle with separation of organic, schizophrenic and neurotic depressions, and also the differentiated approach to the phenomenology of childhood depression in view of the rate of individual physical and mental development (M.G. Usov, 1996), we have conducted research of clinical features of the course of depressive disorders in children.

Analyzing the clinical picture of DN in children, it was found that depressive symptoms in childhood are very rarely stable and form a picture of a complete delineated depressive episode. For the majority of children, variability of symptomatology, saturation by multiple disorders (fragmentary, temporary) are typical, incomplete), combined to form a complex and mosaic picture. When studying clinical types of depression in children without regard to nosological affiliation, the predominant affect in the structure of the depressive syndrome, ideational, motor, behavioral, algic, somatopsychiatric disorders, perceptual disorders, hypochondriacal manifestations, self-blaming ideas, sleep disorders and attraction disorders were studied.

The clinical and psychopathological analysis of the structure of the depressive syndrome allowed to emphasize the general clinical picture of depression and to distinguish psychopathological signs characterizing clinical types of depression in children. As a result of the study, 7 clinical types of the course of MD in children aged 6-14 years were singled out.

The simple clinical type, including ideational disorders manifested by slowness of speech, monosyllabic and long thinking over answers, refusal of game activities requiring mental tension and attention, inability to remember repeatedly re-read material, distraction, difficulty in understanding new material. The decreased mood was characterized by the prevalence of sadness and grief, joylessness and inactivity with a desire for self-isolation, withdrawal. Children stopped to watch their appearance, often cried, were reluctant to leave the house, did not communicate with old friends, stopped being interested in the outside world and did not show interest even in recreational activities. They withdrew into themselves, limiting not only social contacts with peers, but also with relatives, expressing thoughts about their own inadequacy and external unattractiveness.

The vector of guilt in connection with this condition was mainly directed at the parents. A decrease in school progress up to the full refusal of attending school was noted. Children could not explain their unwillingness to study, but often repeatedly said, "I cannot, I do not want to study. Manifestations of the vegetative component of depression were characterized by the disorders of a sleep-wake pattern in the form of a shortening of a night's sleep, difficulties in falling asleep, nightmares and daytime sleepiness. There was an eating disorder, the appetite decreased, children could completely refuse food during the day without a parent's reminder, and if parents insisted, they ate only in small portions, being selective about the food (choosing a sweet or favorite dish). Complaints of palpitations, dizziness, headache or unpleasant bodily sensations in different parts of the body occurred occasionally. Episodes of crying occurred for no apparent reason during the day. Children cried for the slightest reason: at offending, a remark, encouragement, a question, even the appearance of a new thing, etc. Episodic dysphoric-like disorders, provoked by parents' remarks, with motor restlessness, crying, ridiculous threats and actions occurred.

The dysphoric clinical type combines clinical types with a prevalence of resentfulness, irritability and atypical malevolent affect with discontent with others, irritability, irascibility along with ideatorial lethargy and complaints of a "bad", "angry" mood. In general, the mood was gloomy, moody, joyless with absence of pleasure from any kind of activity, dissatisfaction with oneself and others, hostility in combination with reticence and tension. The dominant complaint of children was a feeling of resentment connected with the unjust attitude of others, abandonment. Episodes of crying occurred against a background of irritation, actively expressing ideas of their own unattractiveness. Children committed illegal and aggressive actions directed not only at others, but also at themselves. The reason for hospitalization of the majority of children was a suicide attempt or expressions of suicidal threats or thoughts. Children expressed ideas of their own inadequacy, unattractiveness ("I'm ugly," "I'm stupid," "I'm bad"). The behavior was oppositional, defiant - children damaged their and their parents' belongings, ran away from home, and wandered about. They reacted to the educational measures with irritation, thoughts about injustice of punishment and unappreciation by their parents: "nobody understands me, they don't love me," or with suicidal threats. Children began to smoke, use alcohol, grouped with antisocial adolescents, committed theft both at home and at school, refused to attend or broke discipline at school. Academic performance dropped markedly, fatigue and a pessimistic outlook on life appeared. Children stopped taking care of themselves, did not wash, did not change their clothes. They often ran away from home, wandered about, refused to communicate with peers or were aggressive toward them.

The hypochondriac clinical type included a symptom complex with massive somatoalgic manifestations. Pointing to changes in the child's mental state, parents complained of various body pains or unpleasant sensations with a clear organ projection, or general unpleasant body sensations. General somatic complaints were manifested by headaches, episodes of dizziness, fainting, feeling of weakness, lethargy, chills, sweating, coldness of extremities, subfebrile, low activity of the child. From the gastrointestinal tract, there were complaints of acute abdominal pain, nausea, occasional vomiting, lack of appetite or selectivity in eating. Respiratory system: dyspnea, episodes of choking, episodes of respiratory disorders. Pains ranged from mild, but debilitating, to acute. Cardiovascular system: tachycardia, sensation of cardiac activity interruption. The appearance of the child created a picture of severe physical ailment. These ailments could be either extremely diverse, frequently replacing each other, or, on the contrary, monotonous, limited to one constant complaint. Often children were convinced of an incurable illness. Appetite disorders to the point of refusal to eat were noted in all children. Sleep disturbance in the form of difficulty falling asleep, intermittent, superficial sleep. Children were withdrawn in their worries, isolated from others. They reluctantly went to school or completely refused to study in connection with poor well-being. Episodes of general malaise were interrupted by outbursts of irritability with tears, expressions of thoughts about death. Children lost interest in previous activities or in life completely, were inactive, and spent a long time in bed. Asthenic manifestations prevailed in the first half of the day in the form of weakness, slowness, lethargy, boredom. In the evening, tearfulness, motor restlessness and irritability increased. Children became tearful, constantly tried to draw attention to themselves, expressing ideas of their own unattractiveness. The lowered mood was undifferentiated and masked by the child's general anxiety.

The *anxious-phobic clinical type* united cases with a pronounced display of anxious-phobic symptoms masking existing depressive disorders. The condition was characterized not only by the amplification of "physiological" childhood fears - darkness, loneliness, medical manipulations - but also by the occurrence of fears associated with a feeling of threat to existence (fear of death, physical violence). In other cases, the child's anxiety was heightened with anxious fears covering the habitual vital sphere of the child ("I'm afraid of being beaten at school," "what if there is a war," "how will we live if daddy gets fired"). The child's heightened anxiety was accompanied by the occurrence of episodes of psychomotor anxiety in connection with a change of an external situation (when mother left, when a new person appeared in the house). The vector of anxious fears was directed toward the future and covered the habitual sphere of life of the child (family, school): "what if I do not finish school", "and if my parents die, I will be alone". The refusals to attend school were connected with fears of school, teachers, crowding of children, and answering at the blackboard. In the evening time, there was an amplification of the anxiety component. The fears occurred episodically with verbal agitation, motor overexcitation with stereotypical movements (running in place, moving things around), crying, demanding dissuasion from close relatives. Periodically these states alternated with the affect of melancholy, with complaints about "a sensation of heaviness, a stone on the soul.

Children became withdrawn, tearful, negative, irritable. They often cried, especially in the evening and at night. They complained of "terrible dreams," the contents of which they could not convey. They stopped to aspire to recreational activities - walks, watching cartoons, etc. They reluctantly communicated with peers, expecting danger from them. Becoming apathetic and unconcerned, they aspired to spend more time with parents. The decreased background of mood was represented by sadness, withdrawal, children were lethargic, slow, constantly complained of weariness, sleepiness, refused to communicate and have fun in the company of friends and relatives, reacted poorly to gifts and entertaining events from parents, and were reluctant to leave the house. At the same time, tearfulness was noted, intensifying in the evening.

The *autoaggressive clinical type* included a symptom complex with suicidal tendencies predominating in the depressive symptomatology. The separation of this clinical variant from the dysphoric clinical type is connected with the fact that the child's aggressive behavior was mainly directed at himself or herself in the form of suicide attempts or self-injury. Autoaggressive behavior was manifested by committing single or repeated suicidal acts of pretentious nature (suffocation with pillows, self-hangings on school stairs, pills poisoning, vein dissections, etc.) or self-injuries (tearing out hair and eyebrows, skin cuts, attempts to bang the head against hard objects). Suicide attempts were explained as "unbearable life," "a feeling that they are not understood," bad attitude of peers and parents. Children often cried, blaming the environment for their condition, believing that parents do not love them, "pick on" them, punish them unjustly. These statements were combined with ideas of own unattractiveness ("I am bad", "I am guilty before everyone"). A heavy, gloomy, gloomy mood was accompanied by reticence, tension and hostility, dissatisfaction with myself and others. This condition was accompanied by insomnia, anxiety, a shortening of night sleep and daytime sleepiness. Children had a decreased appetite, up to and including refusal to eat. Refusing to go to school, children hid, and if parents insisted, made suicide attempts at school.

The *regressive clinical type* was defined by the prevalence of mental regression symptoms. This symptom complex is characteristic of all depressive disorders in children. Characteristic for it is the occurrence of regressive (more precisely - pseudo-regressive) disorders, i.e. a return to the forms of behavior and skills peculiar to younger age. Pseudo-regressive disorders in childhood depression were expressed in a temporary suspension of development when for weeks and months, the addition of a vocabulary, acquisition of new motor functions, skills of self-service, more complex forms of play stopped. We observed the occurrence of bedwetting or encopresis in children with already developed self-service skills and the disappearance of these disorders simultaneously with depressive symptoms. There was a change of behavior in the direction of childish forms: aspiration to play with children's toys, occurrence of infantile intonations in speech, slovenliness in dressing and eating, the demand to "take in hands. There was a puerile shade of behavior: imitation in pronunciation of younger children, leering, loss of skills of self-service, loss of the received school knowledge. Children lost the sense of shame, could expose themselves or go to the toilet in front of strangers. Constantly demanded the presence of the mother or the tutor nearby, moved around, holding his or her hand. They refused to go to public institutions by themselves and stayed at home alone. Were afraid to communicate with the surrounding adults and children.

Their school performance decreased markedly, they could not apply the learned knowledge and often refused to go to school. They constantly cried, demanded to see them off in the street. They answered questions out of order. They became overly compassionate - "sorry for the birds who are freezing in the street," "broken toys. Demonstrability, resentfulness, excessive aspiration to cleanliness or, on the contrary, refusal of hygienic procedures appeared in older children. The background of the mood was characterized by dynamism, passivity, slowness, fearfulness. Fears of infantile contents arose: of own death and death of parents, fear of nonexistent events or subjects (Baba Yaga, Bluebeard, Koschey the Immortal, demons, monsters), fear of animals that were not available in our region (a crocodile will eat, a lion will trample a hippo). Children's behavior changed according to these fears: they tried to spend time at home, together with parents, were suspicious of others, reacted negatively to attempts of dissuasion with elements of irritation, ending in tears. Positive emotional events and activities did not provoke an emotional response in them.

The *magiphrenic clinical type* included a symptom complex with changes in the child's behavior directed toward confessional activities: reading religious literature (the Bible, Jehovah's Witnesses literature, etc.), expressing thoughts about the presence of the devil or unclean powers, performing religious rituals, etc. Active cheerful children isolated themselves from the immediate environment, expressed ideas of sinfulness and guilt, and willingly attended confessional events. School maladaptation was manifested by frequent skipping classes or refusing to attend altogether. Children became inactive, aspiring to spend time in seclusion.

The refusal to entertain was explained not only by apathetic manifestations, but also had a self-deprecating character: "I am not worthy. The ideas of own unattractiveness, sinfulness, and thoughts of death were actively expressed. Negativism towards parents manifested itself from the child's expressions of thoughts about their parents' bad or unjust treatment of them to the formation of delusional attitudes in relation to them. Acute psychoproductive disorders in the form of visual and auditory hallucinations and delusions of a demonomaniacal character - voices of the god, the devil, unclean forces, dead relatives "who were calling after them," appearances of people who took away their vital force - were not uncommon. This condition was accompanied by a shortening of night sleep (long falling asleep, shallow sleep or complete insomnia) with nightmares (death, corpses, the dead) and eating disorders (decreased appetite, fasting, selectivity in eating). Mood was sparsely differentiated lowered with constant tearfulness. Children more often named their mood "sad, black, gray, unbearable.

3.1. Clinical features of depression in children with schizophrenia

Investigating depressive disorders in schizophrenia (SD) in children, many authors conclude that these disorders can arise in any age period of childhood in psychopathologically original forms (Iovchuk N.M., Koziulia V.G., 1981; Iovchuk N.M., 1989). G. F. Kolotilin (1971) attributed to the cardinal diagnostic signs of SD, besides monotony of affect, pretentiousness and inadequacy of suicidal actions, the presence of delirium-like fantasizing with elements of pseudo-hallucinations and ideas of influence. H. Remschmidt et al. (1973) noted early signs of schizophrenic psychosis (delusions, symptoms of thought disorder, bipolar mood swings, signs of personality breakdown) in childhood and adolescence, which sometimes go unnoticed because the affective disorders with ideas of sinfulness, remorse, disruption of all activity functions are so lush that they "override" the pathognomonic symptoms for schizophrenia. M.S. Vrono (1973) considered that the most characteristic features of childhood SD are lethargy, moodiness, tearfulness, vegetative disorders, complaints of weakness, vague body discomfort, and also fear, unaccountable anxiety, fear for own life, life and health of relatives, anxiety, quite often accompanied by suicidal tendencies, agitation. W. Spiel (1961) considered empty affect, the predominance in the clinical picture of apathy, fatigue, lethargy, sometimes combined with confusion and anxiety as features of SHD.

A. S. Lomachenkov (1971) described affective disorders in schizophrenia combined with emotional and mental inadequacy, ideatorial-motor dissociation, tension, paradoxicality, unmotivatedness. E.I. Semenovskaya (1972) in periodic schizophrenia in preschool-age children described seizures with predominance of fear, delirium-like fantasies, depressive-delirious, affective-catatonic and affective seizures. Among the features of ASD in children, she names pronounced motor and somatovegetative disorders in the absence of feelings of longing, suicidal tendencies and diurnal mood swings. In children 2-5 years old, dysthymic disorders with irritability, resentment, anger, sleep disorders, fears or adynamy (boredom, lethargy, lack of mobility, lack of interest in the environment), and negativity with resistance, mutism and transient manifestations of regression prevail.

Depressions in children 5-8 years old are more difficult, accompanied by complaints of body discomfort, rudimentary ideas of self-blame, phenomena of mental hyperesthesia. V. N. Mamtseva (1988) described in schizophrenic children of 6-14 years old depressions masked by persistent febrile or pseudoneurological disorders: headaches, dizziness with balance disorder and oculovestibular symptoms combined with depersonalization, derealization and a sense of loss of energy. Despite the phenomenological peculiarity, depression in children is quite comparable to depression in adults. V. M. Bashina (1981) has developed a typology of affective disorders in various forms of the childhood schizophrenic process. In the structure of attack-like schizophrenia with a non-progressive course, six types of depression were singled out: asthenic, mild simple, moody (grumpy), with expressed senestoalgic manifestations, with disorders of self-consciousness, agitated.

The clinical shapes of schizophrenia are acquired by adolescence, allowing dynamic observation and more accurately determine the nosological diagnosis of the disorder. Thus, the average age of the debut of the depressive syndrome in schizophrenia was 11.75 ± 1.8 years and the disorder is predominantly observed in boys, confirming a higher incidence of schizophrenia among this gender (Vrono M. Sch, 1983; Bashina M. V, 1980; Eggers Ch., 1973). Thus, according to H. Stutte (1960), early forms of schizophrenia are observed 3.5 times more often in boys than in girls.

The division into clinical types of depressive states in children is based on the determination of a leading disorder that dominates over other depressive symptomatology and does not disappear during periods of its temporary weakening: the character of the prevailing mood, and in the absence of its differentiation and stability - ideatorial, motor or somatovegetative disorders.

Taking into account the features of the clinical picture, six variants of depression in childhood schizophrenia have been allocated: somatized, magiphrenic, autoaggressive, psychopath-like, simple, anxiously dreary.

The hypochondriacal clinical type of depression in schizophrenia included a symptom complex with massive somatoalgic manifestations. Variants of masked depressions in childhood schizophrenia are of particular importance in the clinic. V. N. Mamtseva (1988), A. A. Severny (1992), I. N. Tatarova (1985), O. D. Sosyukalo (1984), A. A. Kashnikova (1983) describe cases of hyperthermia, vegetovascular disorders and behavioral disorders as "masks". These conditions in some cases masked, in others supplemented the depressive manifestations, unlike masked (vegetative, lavalier) depression. The complex of acute psycho-productive disorders (delusions, hallucinations) was present practically in all cases of observation, but had a touch of somatization. Pointing to changes in the child's mental state, parents complained about various pains or unpleasant sensations of a general somatic character: headaches, episodes of dizziness, fainting states, sensations of weakness, lethargy, low activity of the child.

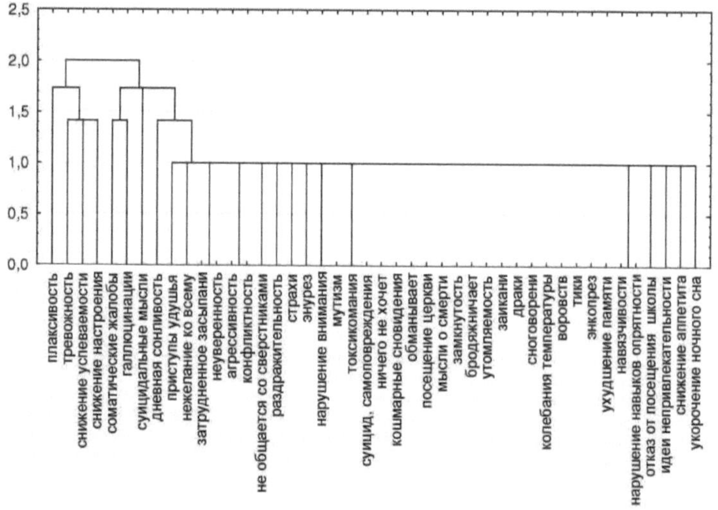

Fig. 16. Cluster analysis of the mental state of children with hypochondriacal type of clinical course of depression on the background of schizophrenia.

Gastrointestinal complaints: acute abdominal pain, nausea, occasional vomiting, lack of appetite or selectivity in eating. Respiratory system: dyspnea, episodes of choking. Pains ranged from mild, but debilitating, to acute, for which the ambulance team was repeatedly called. The duration of the complaints persisted for more than 6 months, the child was repeatedly examined (outpatient and inpatient) by somatic specialists and was treated with vitamin and nootropic drugs without effectiveness. Using the cluster analysis technique, we identified two main clusters of clinical manifestations occurring in these children (Fig. 16).

The <u>somatohypothymic group</u> included complaints of somatic character: palpitations, dizziness, nausea, weakness, sleep disorders, various pains in combination with lethargy ("legs are tired, don't want to walk", "arms and legs are heavy", "it is difficult to walk, I can hardly carry my bag"). The presence of these complaints was combined with a change in the child's appearance and created a picture of a severe physical ailment. These ailments could be either extremely diverse, frequently replacing each other, or, on the contrary, monotonous, limited to one constant complaint. The most frequent complaints in preschool-age children were abdominal pain, and in younger school-age children, headache. Often children were sure that the disease was incurable, even at the mention of someone's illness or death, anxiety increased, and they used in speech medical terms, which included an obvious threat: cancer, AIDS, leprosy, collapse, meningitis, etc. Somatic complaints were accompanied by weak manifestations of hypothymic symptoms in the form of refusal to eat, unsteadiness of mood, tearfulness, refusal of hygienic procedures, sleep disorders. Hallucinatory disorders were predominantly auditory in the form of name-calling, sparse phrases. As a rule, hallucinations were determined at the clinical interview and were the leading factor in the refusal to communicate with the surrounding and close people, children spent a lot of time alone, but preferred not to be alone. If, for some reason, their parents left them, they had anxious states which amplified the depressive symptomatology. The <u>apatoabolic group</u> was defined by complaints of a decrease in the child's activity up to the refusal to attend school or go for walks, desire to spend long hours in bed, inactivity, "lack of interest in life".

The *magifrenic clinical type* of depression in schizophrenia included a symptom complex with a change in the child's behavior directed toward confessional activities (reading religious literature: the Bible, Jehovah's Witness literature, expressing thoughts about the presence of the devil or unclean powers, etc.).

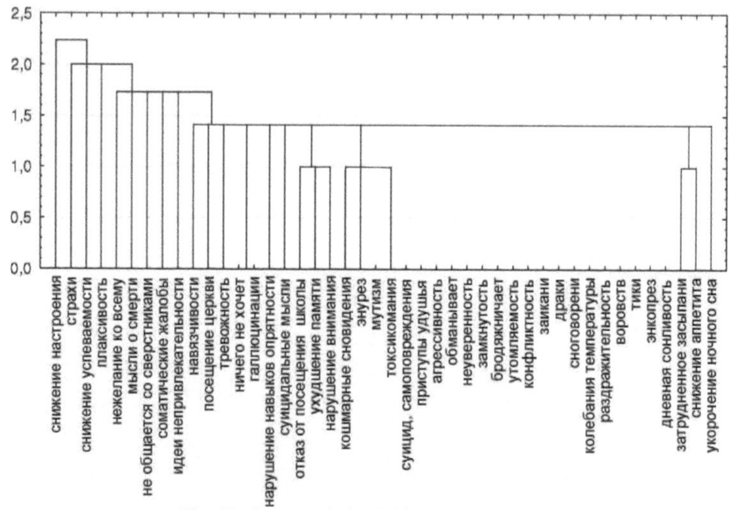

Fig. 17. cluster analysis of children's mental state
with the magiphrenic type of clinical course of depression on the background of
schizophrenia.

Changes in the child's condition were defined by parents as inadequate behavior, with active, cheerful children isolated from the immediate environment, expressing ideas of sinfulness and guilt. Hallucinations in the form of hearing the voice of God or the devil, delusions in relation to relatives or oneself appeared. Using cluster analysis, three main clusters of clinical manifestations were identified (Fig. 17).

The vegetative-religious group was manifested by vegetative manifestations in the form of shortening of night sleep (long falling asleep, shallow sleep or complete insomnia) with nightmares ("death, corpses, dead men") and eating disorders (decreased appetite, fasting, selectivity in eating). Changes in children's behavior were observed with an urge to attend church, a change of clothing style, a demand for baptism, reading of religious literature, performance of religious rituals. The child's behavior was limited to the immediate sphere of life activity (family, school). Children refused to communicate with their peers, but willingly interacted with the people around them during confessional activities. School maladaptation was manifested by frequent absences from school.

Acute psychoproductive disorders in the form of visual and auditory hallucinations and delusions of demonic character - voices of the god, the devil, unclean powers, dead relatives "who were calling after them," appearances of people who took away their vitality were noted. The apathetic group was characterized by inactivity, a desire to spend time in solitude, disinterest in "everything". The refusal to entertain was explained not only by apathetic displays, but also bore a self-deprecating connotation - "I am not worthy. Children actively expressed the ideas of their own unattractiveness, sinfulness, thoughts of death, and presented a large number of health complaints. The hypothymic group was characterized by an undifferentiated lowered mood with constant tearfulness. Children more often named their mood as "black, gray, unbearable," but told little about their experiences to parents. Negativism towards their parents was manifested from the child's expressions of thoughts about their parents' bad or unjust treatment of them to the formation of delirium toward them. As an illustration, we will cite a clinical observation of a patient.

Observat
ion 1

C. A., 11 years old. Admitted for the first time. Complaints on admission: does not sleep well at night (does not fall asleep, wakes up), senses extraneous presence, hears rustles, experiences anxiety. He had no burdened heredity. Lives in the family with the mother and stepfather, child from the mother's first marriage. There is one more daughter by the second marriage, she is healthy. The grandmother on her father's side was notable for her complicated character. The mother is 34 years old, she has higher education, works as a teacher. The father is 42 years old, has secondary technical education, works as a stoker. The child's parents divorced because of the father's complicated character traits (irascibility, inactivity, alcohol abuse). The situation in the family was favorable, and there was a good relationship with the stepfather.

He was born from his first difficult pregnancy. Mother was repeatedly put on the maternity ward. Delivered on time, stimulated. Weight 3100 grams, cried out at once, was attached to the breast in the delivery room. Was not observed by neurologist in the first year of life. The child developed psychomotorally according to his age, started to sit up at 6 months, walk at 11 months, separate words at 1.5 years. The phrasal speech was completely formed by the age of 3. He was silent "not smiling" from an early age. He attended kindergarten from age 3 until school age. He adapted extremely hardly, cried frequently, was "afraid they would forget him in kindergarten," was constantly worried until his mother came. He played little with children and reluctantly participated in matinees. He went to school at 7, following the general education program. He mastered the program well, was indifferent to teaching, had no friends in the class. He is currently studying in the 6th grade. In childhood he had colds, at the age of

4 had episodes of dreaming and dreaming, did not consult doctors, did not get treatment. Denied crashes, seizures, injuries, and operations under general anesthesia. Restless sleep since early childhood. Two months before hospitalization, his condition changed, he was less active, stopped going outdoors and began to study the religious literature available to him. After that, he refused to eat meat ("dead meat"), said there were unclean powers at home, heard rustles and felt that somebody was in the apartment. He insisted on the rite of baptism. During baptism in a monastery, he lost consciousness. After returning home sprinkled holy water on the walls of the house, read a prayer to cast out the unclean spirit. Spends all his time in his room. Since then, he practically stopped sleeping at night and sharply limited his food intake. He drank only water and fasted for two days before being admitted to the hospital. The mother called the child "malocholous.

Somatic condition: normosthenic physique. Skin and visible mucous membranes of normal color. The pharynx was calm. Breathing was vesicular, no rales. The heart tones were clear and rhythmic. The abdomen was soft and painless. The liver and spleen were not enlarged. Physiological excretion was normal. Clinical and biochemical blood tests, general urinalysis without abnormal findings.

Neurological condition: eye slits are the same on both sides, pupils are rounded, reaction to light is preserved. Cranial innervation is not disturbed. The patient confidently performs coordination tests. No sensory disorders were revealed. EEG: moderate diffuse disorganization of bioelectrical activity. No interhemispheric differences or focality. EEG: no pathology.

Mental state: He makes contact, all types of orientation were preserved. The background mood is lowered, anxious, repeatedly looks around, notes that there is a "spirit of evil spirits" in the office. Cannot sleep at night, it seems that there is someone in the room: "the devil is watching me, I see him moving a stool, I hear creaking. When he goes to school, he feels that someone is following him. He is forced to check repeatedly that there is nobody behind him. He is dissatisfied with the situation in the house - "the devil got hold of his stepdad, so he is picky, he curses all the time and he comes in drunk. To protect himself from the devil, he underwent baptism, "but the unclean power was already in me, so I lost consciousness. Emotionally liable, cries. Memory, intellect without gross violations. Thinking is sequential, at a usual pace. During dynamic observation for 64 days, he attended hospital. He brought a Bible, read away from children, refused to eat in the ward, ate only what he blessed at home with holy water and brought with him. He preferred dark-colored clothing, "since I have not yet rid myself of the unclean powers within me. He was anxious.

Diagnosis: schizotypal disorder.

Surveillance analysis: born from the first pregnancy, which proceeded against the background of a constant threat of miscarriage. Formation of mental and locomotor functions took place in usual terms. Developmental dysontogenesis was noted: at the stage of the first age crisis - delayed formation of structures of cognitive and volitional components, dissociative formation of emotional and behavioral components and normal physical development. At the stage of the second age crisis, there was a structural change of the behavioral and affective components in the form of changes in the structure and form of socialization. He was reluctant to communicate with surrounding children, with difficulty adapting in a children's group. He was brought up in a family with an altered structure (by his stepfather), the accepted type of upbringing in the family was "pandering hyperprotection. The child's condition was defined by depressive symptomatology of the magiphrenic type with fragmentary hallucinatory disorders and delirium.

The *autoaggressive clinical type* of depression in SD included a symptom complex with the prevalence of suicidal tendencies in the depressive symptomatology. The separation of this clinical variant from the dysphoric group is related to the fact that aggressive behavior was predominantly self-directed in the form of suicide attempts or self-harm. Although schoolchildren distinguished between the concepts of life and death, death was estimated by them as a temporary phenomenon. Almost all girls from the age of 12 years and boys from the age of 15 years understood the finality of their own lives and experienced it, however only 20.0% of teenagers realized that death is the final termination of physical and spiritual life (Isaev D.N., 1993).

In our research sample, children did not reach the necessary age period and committing suicide attempts or self-harm were associated with the presence of DR. Parents noticed changes in the child's condition due to the appearance of a reduced mood, tearfulness, refusal of hygiene procedures, irritability arising when parents tried to clarify the situation, expressing thoughts of not wanting to live, self-injury or suicide attempts. Using the cluster analysis technique, we identified three main clusters of clinical manifestations (Fig. 18).

The hypothymic group was expressed by vegetative manifestations in the form of insomnia, anxiety, shorter nighttime sleep, and daytime sleepiness. Children had a decreased appetite, up to and including refusal to eat. Children often cried, blaming their environment for their condition, believing that parents did not love them, "pick on" them, punish them unjustly. These statements were combined with ideas of own unattractiveness ("I am bad", "I am guilty before everybody"). Heavy, gloomy, gloomy mood was accompanied by withdrawal, tension, hostility, dissatisfaction with themselves and others. Children actively expressed suicidal ideas. They refused to go to school, hid if parents insisted, and made suicide attempts at school.

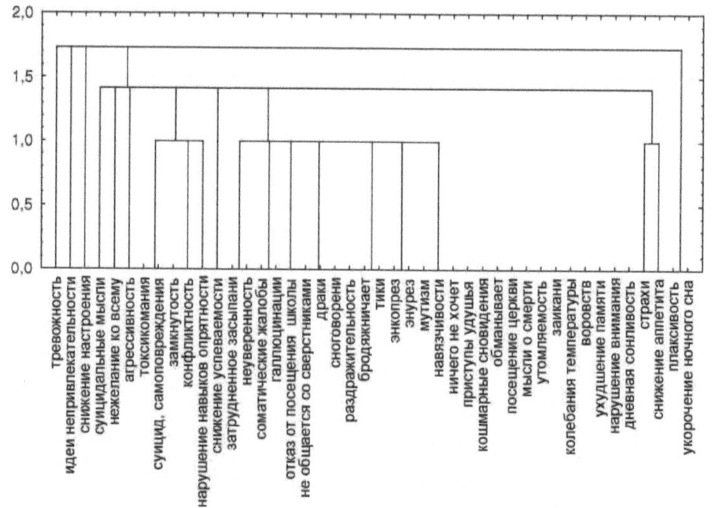

Figure 18. Cluster analysis of children's mental state
with autoaggressive type of clinical course of depression on the background of schizophrenia.

The psychopathic group was characterized by outbursts of rage, rudeness and swearing at close relatives. Episodes of irritability alternated with tearfulness and depression. Children aspired to leave home, vagabonded, joined antisocial personalities and refused to communicate with former friends.

The auto-aggressive group was manifested by committing single or repeated suicidal acts, which were of pretentious character, or by self-inflicted injuries. Suicide attempts were explained by "unbearable life", "feeling that they are not understood", bad attitude of peers and parents. As an illustration, we will cite a clinical observation of a patient.

Dysphoric clinical type   Change of state were characterized mainly by rudeness, insolence, spitefulness, aggressiveness, increased excitability, despotism, combined with behavioral disorders: skipping classes, refusal to attend school, fighting, anti-disciplinary behavior, vagrancy. Using the cluster analysis technique, we identified an overall cluster of clinical manifestations, divided into two main subgroups (Fig. 19).

The first subgroup of the altered mental condition was represented by behavioral disorders of a psychopath-like character. Children became conflictual and aggressive in relation to close relatives, friends and pets, and expressed fragmented delusional ideas of the attitude of their closest environment. An overwhelming hostile attitude toward the closest people, most often mothers, was observed. Outbursts of rage with pugnacity and spite were noted, at these moments, they could inflict heavy physical harm on others. When leaving home, they began to vagabond, drink alcoholic beverages. When going to school, they showed aggression in relation to their classmates, to remarks they reacted violently negatively, and they spent time in lessons passively. However, they rarely refused to go to school.

The second group was represented by the manifestations characterized by a lowered mood, verbalized as heavy, gloomy, sullen. Children were always dissatisfied with something, withdrawn, grumpy, unavailable. They were dissatisfied with all kinds of activities, even those which they loved before. They readily fantasized about death, but did not express suicidal intentions. There was a slight change of appetite in the direction of consumption of favorite dishes and refusal of the rest. Sleep disorders were manifested mainly by difficulties in falling asleep and the presence of nightmares of sadistic or sexual nature. Ideas self-abasement and self-blame were sporadic in the form of episodic statements about their own inadequacies.

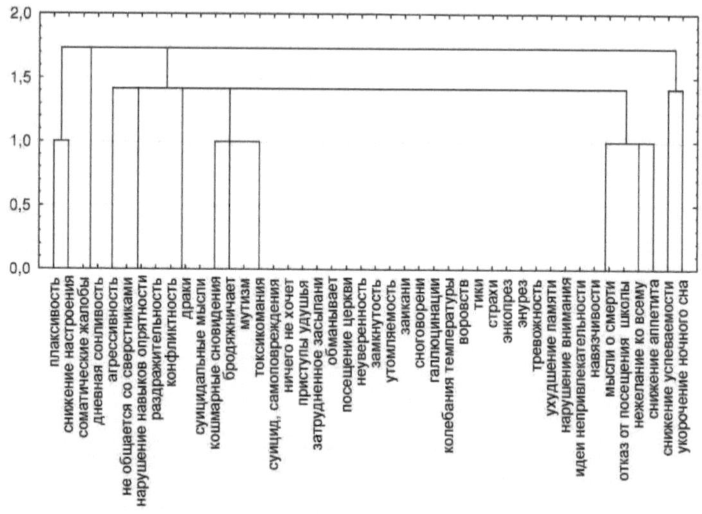

Fig. 19. cluster analysis of the psychological state of children with a dysphoric type of clinical course of depression against a background of schizophrenia.

The simple clinical type of childhood SD depression combined clinical types with a prevalence of undifferentiated lowered mood, sadness, and sadness accompanied by lowered self-esteem and pessimistic assessment of the present and future. Parents complained of sadness and sadness in their children, accompanied by low self-esteem and a pessimistic assessment of the present and future.

Children were depressed, joyless, complained of boredom, desire to cry for no reason. Pleasant events did not cause a vivid emotional reaction, while insignificant external negative factors significantly worsened well-being and mood. Using the technique cluster analysis technique, we identified one general cluster of clinical manifestations (Fig. 20).

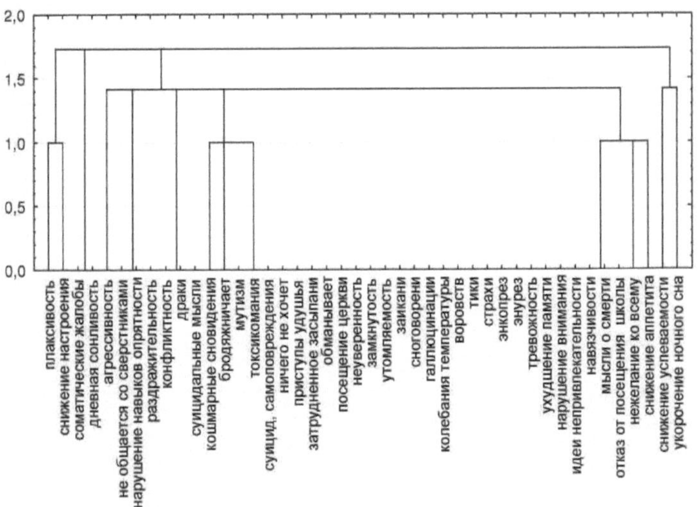

Fig. 20. cluster analysis of the mental state of children with a simple type of clinical course of depression on the background of schizophrenia.

The most vivid were ideatorial disorders manifested in the form of slowness of speech, monosyllabic and long thinking over answers, refusal of play activity requiring mental tension and attention, inability to remember repeatedly read material, distraction, difficulty in assimilating new material. As a consequence, there was a pronounced decrease in the child's academic performance and a refusal to give oral answers at school. The lowered mood was characterized by sadness and sadness, joylessness and inactivity. Children were reluctant to go out, did not communicate with former friends, and expressed ideas of their own inconsistency, squalor, and external unattractiveness. The vector of blame was mainly directed on parents: "We do not have enough money", "It's your fault that I am so ugly. Episodes of crying occurred for no apparent reason during the day, cried for the slightest reason: at the slightest offence, a remark, encouragement, a question, etc. They hardly fell asleep and refused to eat. Episodic dysphoric-like disorders, provoked by parents' remarks, with motor restlessness, crying, ridiculous threats and actions.

The *anxious-phobic clinical type* of depression in schizophrenia was characterized by the prevalence of anxious-tosickly symptoms. Anxiety prevailed in parents' complaints about their children's condition: children would not be left alone at home, would not let their parents go, were fearful of interacting with peers.

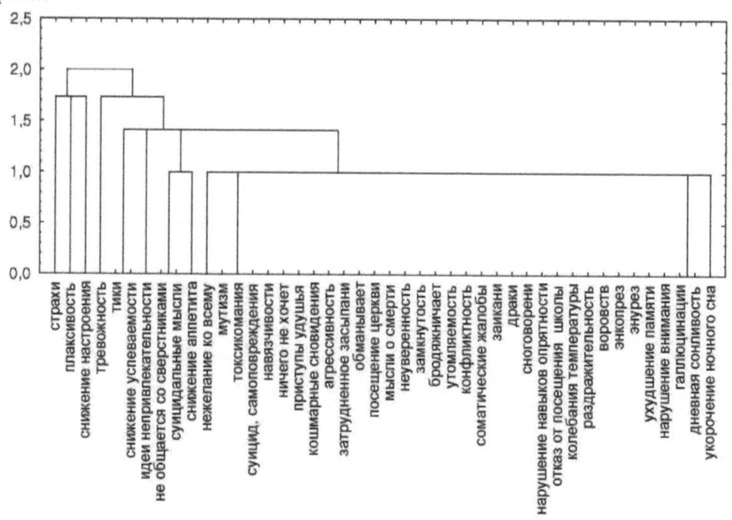

Fig. 21. cluster analysis of children's mental state
with the anxious-phobic type of the clinical course of depression on the background of schizophrenia.

Periodically this condition alternated with the affect of melancholy, with complaints of "a feeling of heaviness, a stone on the soul," motor overexcitation with stereotypical movements (running in place, moving things). Children became withdrawn, tearful, negative, irritable. Using the cluster analysis technique, we identified two main clusters of clinical manifestations (Fig. 21).

The hypothymic group was manifested by the vegetative component of depression in the form of sleep disturbance and eating disorders. The decreased background of mood was represented by sadness and withdrawnness. Children were lethargic, slow, lethargic, constantly complaining of fatigue, sleepiness. They refused to communicate and have fun with friends and relatives. They reacted poorly to gifts and entertainment from parents, and were reluctant to leave the house. Tearfulness was noted, intensifying by the evening, accompanied by short episodes of agitation with discontinuous hallucinatory disorders.

The neurotic group was manifested by heightened anxiety with the occurrence of episodes of psychomotor anxiety in connection with a change of the external situation (when the mother left, when a new person appeared in the house). The vector of anxious fears was directed on the future and covered the habitual sphere of life of the child (family, school): "What if I will not finish school", "and if parents die, I will remain alone". On a background of general uneasiness, there were pretentious fears (of vampires, nuclear war). The fears arose episodically with verbal agitation, tears, and demands for dissuasion from close relatives. The fears, acquiring a fanciful plot, were accompanied by deceptions of perception (sketchy visual and auditory hallucinations in the form of rustles, breathing, shadows or with formed figurative hallucinations - monsters, spirits), a sense of extraneous presence. Against a background of fears, children formed ritual actions involving their immediate environment.

**3.2. Clinical features of the course of depressive
mood disorders
in children of neurotic nature**

Much less works are devoted to the problem of neurotic depression (ND) in children than in adults. However, a sufficient number of works of domestic and foreign researchers (A.E. Lichko, 1979; Sinytsky, 1979; Sinytsky, 1979) are devoted to the description of a clinical and psychological picture of ND in adolescence, their diagnostics and differential diagnostics. E., 1979; Sinitsky V. N., 1986; Podkorytov V. S. et al., 1989; Nissen G., 1977; Winokur O. T., 1987; Lewinsohn P. M. et al., 1995). Y. A. Makarenko (1977) considered signs of PND in children as tension, anxiety, restlessness, difficulty in speaking, infantile behavior, lack of appetite, nightmares, pathological habits such as finger sucking or nail biting. Я. P. Girich (1970), describing depressive reactions in children after heavy mental trauma (death and illness of relatives), allocated a gradual decrease in the background mood with loss of motor activity and play interest. Children became tearful, depressed, and their sleep and appetite worsened. Subsequently, this background was accompanied by asthenoneurotic disorders: fatigue, irritability, enuresis, tics, fears, etc. According to some authors (V.M. Kozidubova, 1992; H.S. Akiskal, 1983; D. Marcelli, 1995, etc.), the clinic of VD has considerable distinctions in different age periods. More typical manifestations close to the symptomatology of non-psychotic depression in adults are observed in puberty and partially - in prepuberty age.

Thus authors allocate the following clinical features: the expressed dependence on a psychotraumatic situation, experience of dissatisfaction of the attitude of parents, abundance of somatovetegetative disorders and violations of behavior in the form of situational personal reactions of protest, refusal, hypercompensation, emancipation which are quite often accompanied by asocial and even delinquent behavior (vagrancy, theft, alcoholism, etc.). T.B. Dmitrieva (1981), studying neurotic episodes in teenagers, marked the originality of affective displays in the period of puberty: considerable expression of vegetative and neurotic disorders, neurotic level of disorganization of mental activity, atypicality of actually depressive

symptomatology, inclusion of specific adolescent behavioral reactions in the clinical picture. The most delineated ND in adolescents are described by forensic psychiatrists (Natalievich E.S. et al., 1982; Posokhova V.I., 1982).

From the variety of clinical variants of ND existing in psychiatric practice, the authors allocate the following in teenagers: asthenic, anxious, dysphoric, hysterical, hypochondriac. On the basis of clinical and psychopathological features, Y.F. Antropov (2001) defined typological variants of ND: anxious, asthenic, asthenic-disturbed and anxiously-disturbed. In characterizing ND in children and teenagers, N.V. Rimashevskaya (1999) mentions only some of its signs: depression occurs in conditions of emotional deprivation and is characterized by bawdiness, moodiness, sleep disorders, anorexia or bulimia, sometimes with regression of behavior and loss of skills acquired earlier, i.e. affective pathology is spoken about too briefly, as if to imply its presence in the structure of other disorders.

This clinical variant of neurotic depression combines clinical types with a prevalence of resentfulness, irritability with dissatisfaction with others, irascibility along with ideatorial retardation, committing illegal and aggressive actions directed not only at others, but also at themselves. Taking into account the features of the clinical picture, four clinical variants of neurotic and cyclical depressive disorders in children are allocated: dysphoric, hypochondriacal, simple, anxious-phobic.

Dysphoric clinical type of depression. The reason for hospitalization of half of the children in this group was a suicide attempt (more often in the form of drug poisoning) or the expression of suicidal threats or thoughts. However, even in these cases, hospitalization was not an emergency; the children were admitted as planned. On admission, parents complained about the child's passivity, alternating with episodes of psychomotor agitation, auto-aggressive statements, desire to run away from home, general negativism directed at himself (dissatisfaction with his physical appearance or mental abilities) or at others (refusal to communicate with peers, lack of interest in life). School maladaptation in the form of reduced academic performance or complete refusal to answer in class or attend school, alcohol consumption or smoking is characteristic. Using the cluster analysis technique, we identified three main clusters of clinical manifestations (Fig. 22).

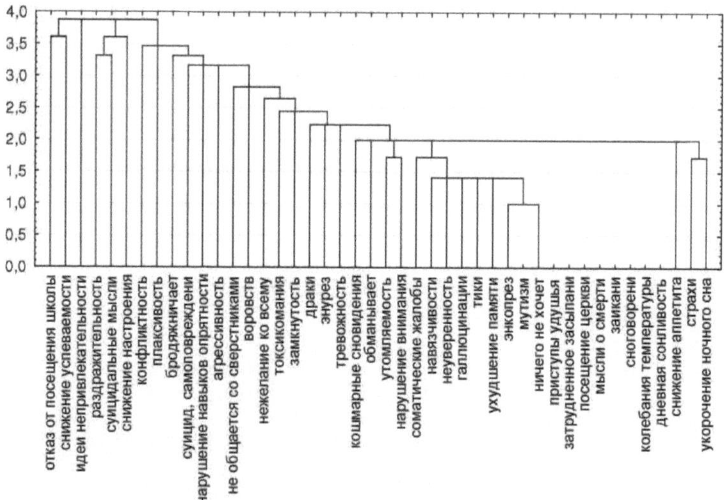

Fig. 22. cluster analysis of mental state in children with a dysphoric type of clinical course of depressive disorder.

The <u>asthenoneurotic group</u> was characterized by idealotor retardation with refusal to engage in favorite activities and communicate with friends. Children became insecure, often complained of fatigue, weakness, body discomfort, lack of appetite and feeling of rest after a night's sleep, and unpleasant dreams. Academic problems were explained by poor memory ("I cannot remember what I said at school," "I cannot concentrate on the task") and a lack of interest in learning. In some cases, children had intrusive movements.

The <u>psychopathic group</u> was characterized by oppositional defiant behavior with discontent directed against themselves and their relatives. Children told invented unpleasant stories about their parents, expressed ideas of their own inadequacy, unattractiveness ("I am ugly," "I am stupid," "I am bad"). They stopped taking care of themselves, did not wash, did not change their clothes. They often ran away from home, vagranted, began to drink or smoke, or stole money from their parents. They refused to communicate with peers or were aggressive with them. If irritability was pronounced, they began to threaten to commit suicide or inflict self-injury. The hypotymic-dysphoric group was characterized by a lowered mood with apathy, resentfulness, negativism to inquiries, and general conflictedness. The mood was described by children as "black, angry. School maladaptation was manifested by the refusal to attend school and a negative attitude toward learning, a pronounced decrease in academic achievement.

The hypochondriac clinical type of depression combined cases with an abundance of hypochondriacal complaints simulating somatic disorders. The sharp change of the child's condition with apathy, tearfulness, indifference to the surrounding world attracted the attention of parents. Together with these symptoms, children complained of painful unpleasant sensations in the body, which had clear localizations ("a lump in the throat," "a stone in the stomach," "the legs fall off").

Behavior changed according to the available symptoms, for example, children refused to take solid food or completely refused to eat. In some cases, the child's condition mimicked a somatic disorder without clear localization of symptoms. There was a prolonged slight increase in temperature (up to 37.1-37.3 ° C). Children were lethargic, joyless, apathetic to the world around, and spent a lot of time in bed. In connection with these complaints, some parents sought examination by pediatricians and underwent in-patient examination. The treatment received did not lead to a change in the condition, so they sought help from a psychiatrist. Using the cluster analysis technique, we identified two main clusters of clinical manifestations (Fig. 23).

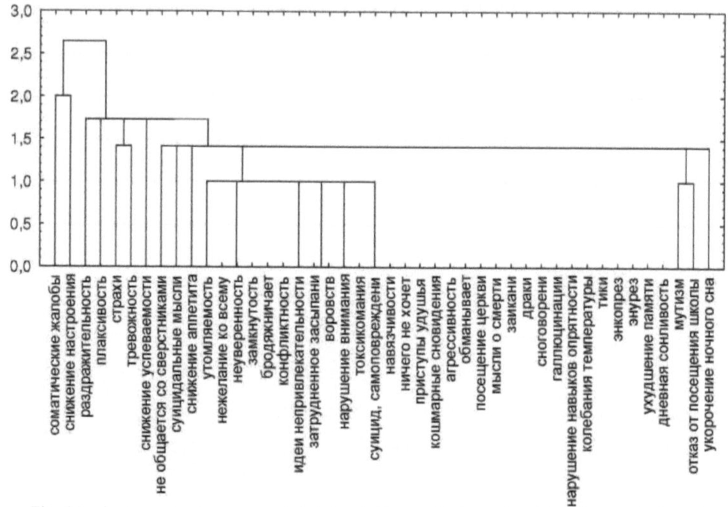

Fig. 23. cluster analysis of mental state in children with hypochondriacal type of clinical course of depressive disorder.

The <u>vegetative group</u> was characterized by disturbed nighttime sleep in the form of difficulty falling asleep, short duration, restlessness with frequent awakening and crying, lack of feeling of rest, sleepiness during the day, eating disorders in the form of selective eating or complete absence of appetite, signs of physical malaise (subfebrile fever, chills, sweating, cold extremities, tachycardia, abdominal pain, lump in the throat, headaches, seizures of respiratory disorders). Somatic complaints were accompanied by general adynamy, ideas of own insolvency. Children refused to communicate with parents and peers, expressed ideas of their own death, imagined their own funerals. Episodically the statements had suicidal overtones: "I'd rather die," "I don't want to live like that.

The <u>hypothymic hypochondriac group was characterized by</u> low-differentiated lowered mood and general anxiety, occurrence of fragmentary fears about own life and health and about health of close relatives ("I will die", "I have cancer"), fears about the future. Episodic episodes of irritability occurred, directed at oneself, with tears and speech agitation. The ideas of own unattractiveness were constantly expressed. Children did not refuse to attend school, but had difficulties in their oral responses up to and including loss of active speech, were excessively anxious about their grades, and had a hard time learning the curriculum.

The *anxious-phobic clinical type* of depression included cases of MD with a pronounced manifestation of anxious-tosickly symptoms, masking the existing depressive disorders. The change of a condition was characterized by sudden occurrence of the fears connected with sensation of threat in usual areas of life activity (fears for life and health of their parents, about their own safety), or by the increase of the general alarming background. Children often cried, especially in the evening and at night. They complained of "terrible dreams," the contents of which they could not convey. They stopped to aspire to entertainments - walks, watching cartoons, etc. They reluctantly communicated with peers, expecting from this communication to be threatening. They became apathetic, apathetic, and tried to spend more time with parents. They refused to go to school in connection with their fears of teachers, crowds of children, answers at the blackboard.

Based on these complaints, parents sought help from child psychologists and psychotherapists. However, there was no effectiveness against the background of the No treatment was observed, and the condition of the children remained unchanged or worsened. Using the cluster analysis technique, we identified three main clusters of clinical manifestations (Fig. 24).

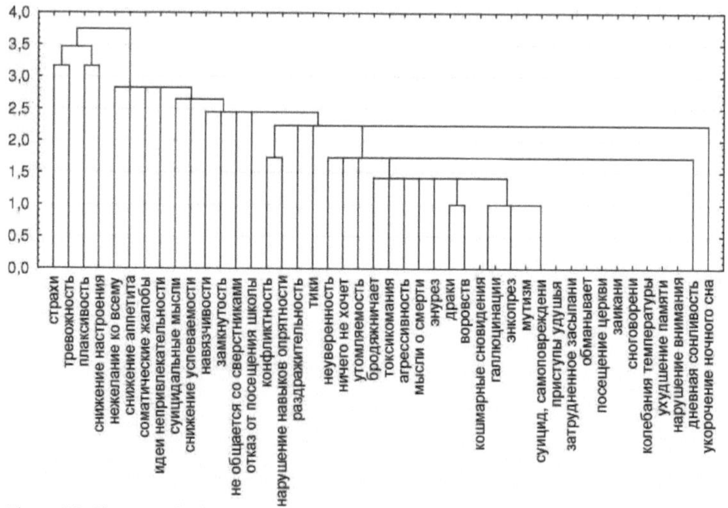

Figure 24. Cluster analysis of mental state in children with the anxious-phobic type of clinical course of depressive disorder.

The <u>dysphoric group</u> was characterized by episodic attacks of motor and speech agitation with irritability, tears, complaints about the state of health and desire to injure oneself or others. These attacks were usually initiated by the desire of parents to involve the child in family or school affairs. Ideas of self-blame, limited to family and school problems, combined with ideas of abandonment, unfairness of the offenses inflicted and self-pity were actively expressed. Some children tended to run away from home during such attacks.

The <u>hypotymic-anxiety group</u> manifested itself as a lowered mood *with* refusal to communicate with peers, reticence, expressing ideas of their own unattractiveness. Children expressed doubts concerning parental love, became withdrawn, inactive, refused to eat, reacted poorly to parents' efforts to please or entertain. However, they aspired to be constantly in the apartment together with close people, expressing anxious fears if any of relatives did not return home on time. The <u>hypotymic-phobic group</u> was characterized not only by an increase in "physiological" childhood fears - darkness, loneliness, medical manipulation, but also by the appearance of fears connected with a feeling of threat to existence (fear of death, physical violence). In other cases, there was an increase in the child's fearfulness with anxious fears covering the habitual sphere of life ("I'm afraid of being beaten at school," "what if there is a war," "how will we live if daddy gets fired").

The simple clinical type of depression combined ND with an undifferentiated lowered mood, the prevalence of sadness and grief, pessimistic assessment of the present and the future, and lowered self-esteem. Complaints of sad mood, pessimistic thoughts, lack of interest in life, general passivity, and tearfulness. Some parents sought outpatient care from pediatricians and received general restorative treatment (vitamins, nootropic and vascular medications). However, against the background of treatment, the condition remained unchanged, children were still indifferent, did not communicate with other children, and were reluctant to attend school, explaining that they "did not want to see anyone. Using the cluster analysis technique, we identified two main clusters of clinical manifestations (Fig. 25).

The vegetative-dysphoric group was manifested by the vegetative component of depression in the form of disorders of night sleep (insomnia and nightmares), daytime sleepiness, decreased appetite, complaints of asthenic content: constant fatigue, pronounced fatigability, painful sensations in the body without certain localization. Children willingly talked about death, changing the phablet of the conversation from conditional desirability ("death is better than such a life", "I want to die as my mother") to fearfulness in connection with its possible occurrence.

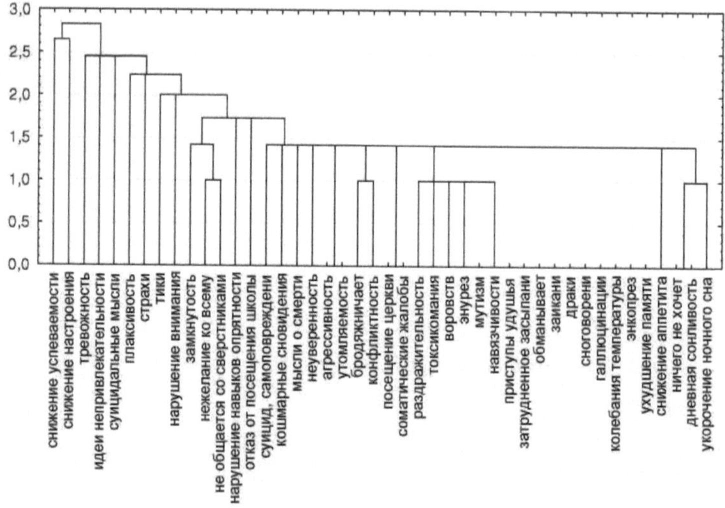

Fig. 25. cluster analysis of mental state in children with a simple type of clinical course of depressive disorder.

The dysphoric component was manifested in the commission by the child of thefts with the subsequent expenditure of money for entertainment and outbursts of irritability with a vector directed toward relatives. The hypothetical group was characterized by a lowered mood of the child with the desire for self-isolation and isolation. Children stopped attending to their appearance and often cried. There was a decrease in school performance up to and including a complete refusal to attend school. Children could not explain their unwillingness to study, but often repeatedly said, "I cannot, I do not want to study. Against this background

The condition actively expressed suicidal thoughts.   As

To illustrate, here is a clinical observation of a patient.

Observation 3

P. M., 12 years old. Comes in for the first time. Complains of fatigue, headaches, adynamia ("can lie in bed all day"), tearful, refuses to do homework, go to school, does not talk to parents and friends.

Heredity: the mother's brother has schizophrenia. Mother is 43 years old, has higher education, works in her field of study. Describes herself as impressionable and insecure. Father is 50 years old, higher education, works as a trainer in another city. The parents of the child have been divorced for 10 years, the boy has no contact with his biological father. The mother was remarried, the child had been living with his stepfather for 2.5 years, the child was from his second marriage, and he was healthy. Relationships in the family are dysfunctional, the stepfather abuses alcohol, and there are constant quarrels and scandals at home.

The child was born from the 4th pregnancy, first delivery at the age of 31. All previous pregnancies ended in miscarriages. Pregnancy was perilous and the mother had several miscarriages. Caesarean section delivery, weight at birth - 3250 grams, Apgar score 7/8. The baby was attached to the breast on the third day. The child was discharged from the maternity hospital with the diagnosis: "Hip joint dyskinesia". Formation of mental and locomotive functions in accordance with normal physiological development. Was observed by a neurologist due to the fact that he did not sleep well at night, was tearful and sleepy during the day. He was diagnosed with perinatal encephalopathy and received no treatment. Up to 6 years old, he did not attend preschool and was brought up at home by his grandmother. He was active, active, willingly communicated with peers. From the age of 6, he spent some time in preschool, because he was often ill with infectious diseases. He started going to school at the age of 8 (kindergarten school), with the 1:4 program, mastered the program well, went to school willingly, had many friends. His mother characterized the child as withdrawn and quiet. In his free time, he is fond of computer games.

He denied any traumatic brain injury, seizures, dreaming, sleepwalking. At the age of 3.4, he had laryngotracheitis, for which he was treated in a children's hospital. At the age of 10, a speech therapist diagnosed him with dyslalia. Observed by a pediatrician with the diagnosis: chronic tonsillitis; abnormal chord of the left ventricle; biliary dyskinesia. At the age of 9, he had chicken pox.

The condition first changed after the birth of his brother at the age of 8 years, relations with his stepfather worsened sharply, he became irritable, reluctant to communicate with relatives, spent much time in bed, sleep and appetite were disturbed. He did not consult any specialists with these complaints, his condition normalized within a month. Condition changed about 4 months ago due to constant scandals in the family. He became withdrawn, "quiet," refused to go outside, spent most of the time at home, "at the window, waiting for his father. A lowered mood was noted. A month before hospitalization, his appetite decreased, he had difficulty falling asleep in the evening, "could fall asleep at 4-5 in the morning. He constantly complained of fatigue, headaches, began to miss school and "could not do homework. When he was involved in recreational activities (a trip to the circus), he stopped talking to parents, hid under a blanket and did not want to see anybody. If they tried to force-feed the child, he would scream and cry. Two weeks before hospitalization, the parents consulted a neurologist with these complaints.

At the doctor's appointment he did not speak, and after the appointment he tried to run away from his parents, screaming and crying, due to which his mother called an ambulance and a shot of Sibazon was given.

The neurologist prescribed treatment with Sonapax in a dose of 30 mg per day, but no efficacy of treatment was noted. We went to a psychiatrist on our own.

Somatic condition: the condition is satisfactory, the physique is correct, asthenic. Skin, pharynx, visible mucous membranes were pale pink, clean. Vesicular breathing, no rales on auscultation. The heart tones were clear and rhythmic. The abdomen was soft, painless, liver and spleen were not enlarged. Clinical and biochemical blood tests, general urinalysis without abnormal findings.

Neurological condition: eye slits are the same on both sides, pupils are rounded, reaction to light is preserved. Cranial innervation is not impaired. Tendon reflexes are evoked in full volume, on both sides. The patient confidently performs coordination tests. No sensitivity disorders were revealed. EEG, REG without pathology.

Mental state: He comes into contact, is aloof in conversation, reluctant to talk about his condition. During the conversation, he complains about his parents, "They make me eat," "I want to be alone, but they don't let me. He characterizes his mood as bad, "on the three-point mark. He said that at night he had scary dreams about death and sometimes had pessimistic thoughts, denying suicidal thoughts. Denies hallucinations, does not detect behavior, no delusional statements. The rate of mental performance is slower. Attention is difficult to concentrate. Thinking at a slower pace. Formal, detached, emotionally inexpressive. Intelligence within the age norm. Denies fears and anxiety. Appearance of depression on the Hamilton scale corresponds to 19 points, on the Kovacek school - 15 points. The child's social age corresponds to 11 years old. During dynamic observation, the child regularly visited the hospital, communicated little with the children. He spent his time without any activity. He did not attend school lessons. Often cried for no apparent reason, complained of headaches and weakness. He was treated with 50 mg of Stimuloton per day, during treatment his mood improved, he began to communicate with children around him, willingly attended classes at school, his appetite leveled off, his sleep improved.

Diagnosis: "Depressive behavioral disorder.

Observation analysis: impairment of social development was observed, he was brought up in a family with an altered structure (stepfather), a pathological type of upbringing was revealed in the family: "hyperopedding", he did not attend preschool. On a background of a chronic psychotraumatic situation (constant scandals in the family), reactive depression (simple clinical type) was observed

3.3. Clinical features of the course of depressive mood disorders in children with mental retardation

Studies concerning depressive disorders in children with mental retardation (DRD) are extremely scarce. Conducting studies among mentally retarded children - students of correctional schools and boarding schools in Moscow, V.V. Konovalova, T.A. Kupriyanova, T.N. Prilepskaya (2004) revealed that the prevalence of depression is 7.6% among all students. According to their research, girls with mental retardation are more likely to be depressed than boys. N.A. Bohan, N.E. Butorina, E.N. Krivulin (2006), studying depressive reactions in penitentiary maladjustment in adolescents, also revealed ODD. Common variants of the depressive reaction for all mentally retarded adolescents were asthenoapathic and dysphoria-like. For mentally retarded individuals with substance dependence, an anxious version of the depressive response was identified. Obsessive-phobic, hypochondriacal and delinquent versions of depression are typical for mentally retarded adolescents without signs of substance dependence. Manifestations of depression in oligophrenia are atypical by the clinic and by the course. The basic symptomatology of oligophrenia is quite brightly revealed both in the content of psychotic experiences and in a certain specificity of psychopathological syndromes. The elementary nature of psychopathological manifestations is characteristic.

Many patients have somatoneurological signs in the clinical structure of psychosis in the form of headaches, dizziness, sleep disorders, acute fatigue and exhaustion. Depressive states are usually superficial, characterized by a monotonous lowered mood with a dysphoric or dysthymic tone. Quite often depressive episodes are accompanied by anxiety, undifferentiated fears, nervousness and confusion. Some children with shallow intellectual defects reveal unsteady, unformed ideas of treatment and self-blaming: patients consider themselves "bad", "fools", they feel that they are looked at and sometimes suicidal behavior is possible. An abundance of hypochondriacal statements and senestopathies is characteristic. Hypochondriac complaints are characterized by polymorphism, variability, fluctuations in intensity and pathological sensations. In their contents, they are simple, primitive, concrete and are often accompanied by a search for help from others. Complaints are presented in the form of annoying clinginess, lamentations (V. V. Kovalev, 1995).

Taking into account the features of the clinical picture, three variants of depression in children with mental retardation were allocated: simple, dysphoric, regressive.

The simple clinical type of depression combined typological variants characterized by slightly differentiated lowered mood with manifestations of motor and ideational retardation, but without prevalence of somatogegetative and neurological manifestations of depression. In the anamnesis some of the children had a diagnosis of "oligophrenia" (F70.0) and underwent a correctional program. In all cases, the diagnosis was made on an outpatient basis, and the corrective form of education was recommended by the medical-pedagogical commission.

All patients consulted a psychiatrist for the first time with complaints of a change in their condition.

Parents complained about a pronounced decrease in the child's progress in both remedial and general education programs. Children refused to attend school, orally answered lessons, did homework, and expressed pessimistic thoughts. When trying to stimulate learning, they complained of headaches and fatigue. In addition, children were tearful and touchy regardless of the situation. Children lost interest in the world around them, showing no interest even in recreational activities. They withdrew into themselves, limiting not only social contacts with peers, but also with relatives, trying to spend time alone. Verbal activity decreased, and there was a decrease in emotional resonance. Children became slow, withdrawn, "as though submerged in their own thoughts. In some cases, nighttime sleep was reduced. Using the cluster analysis technique, we identified two main clusters of clinical manifestations and additional groups of psychiatric symptoms that had weak statistical correlations with other psychiatric symptoms, and consequently, were not grouped together (Fig. 26).

The hypothymic group included the lowered mood of the child with tearfulness on any occasion, detachment. Children expressed pessimistic thoughts about the future and the present, but these statements were of a primitively infantile character. Often they withdrew into their experiences, not verbalizing them. Such children did not communicate at school with peers and younger children, the play interests previously peculiar to them disappeared. There was a breach of neatness skills: the ability to dress, eat and use hygienic procedures independently decreased. Children had difficulties mastering curriculum material in schools, which strengthened the manifestations of depressive disorders.

The vegetative group included manifestations of the vegetative component of depression in the form of changes in night sleep (more often excessive sleepiness at night and during the day), decreased appetite, hypochondriacal complaints (fatigue, headaches, abdominal pain, difficulty breathing, without clear localization). In some cases, mild subfebrile fever (up to 37.0-37.2 ° C) was noted. Among the individual symptoms, irritability, tendency to minor conflicts with peers, and inactivity were quite common.

The *dysphoric clinical type* of depression united cases of DP with prevailing behavioral disorders in children. In all cases, the diagnosis was made on an outpatient basis, the corrective form of education was recommended by the medical-pedagogical commission. Parents or guardians of the child presented complaints about early alcoholization, tobacco smoking, substance abuse, propensity to vagrancy or running away, theft.

Children were dissatisfied with their parents' attitude toward them, considering them guilty of poor health, expressing a lot of claims and reproaches; were aggressive in relation to relatives or small children (beatings, threatening with a knife or other subjects). Quite often, there were auto-aggressive manifestations: threatening to commit suicide, self-traumatization, and suicide attempts. At school, pronounced disorders of Conduct leading to conflicts with teachers and surrounding children. Often children refused to further attend school, spending time in the company of peers with anti-disciplinary behavior. The clustering procedure identified two subgroups from the general cluster of mental disorders in this type of depression (Fig. 27).

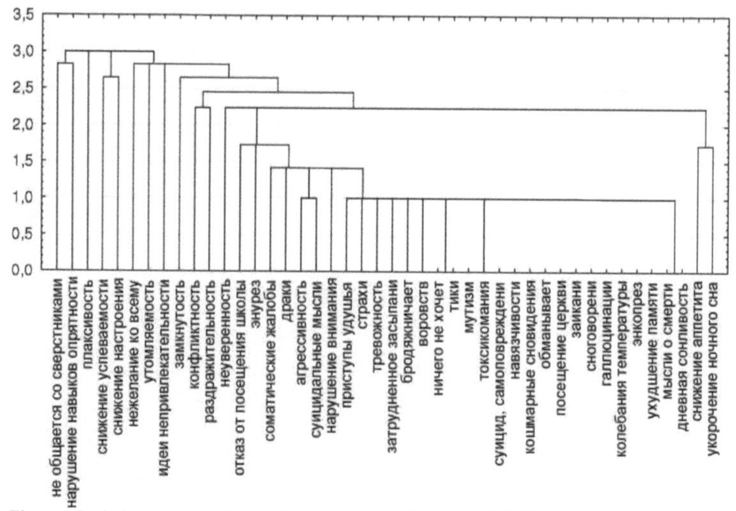

Figure 26. cluster analysis of mental status in mentally retarded children with a simple type of clinical course of depressive disorder.

Reduced mood with a touch of dysphoria, ideas of general unattractiveness ("Yes, I am bad, but I will be even worse," "I know that it is bad, but it is easier for me"), reticence (children were reluctant to reveal their experiences, had little contact with peers and adults) dominated among manifestations of hypothymic symptoms.

There was a disturbance of night sleep, mainly in the form of insomnia. In the general negativism facet, children stopped washing themselves and using toiletries. They often expressed suicidal thoughts, willingly told how their body would look after death, bequeathed their belongings. In a number of cases, suicide attempts were observed. Psychopathic manifestations ranged from general negativism, threats to close people, destruction of personal belongings or school textbooks to beatings of children, peers or elderly people and threats to kill close people.

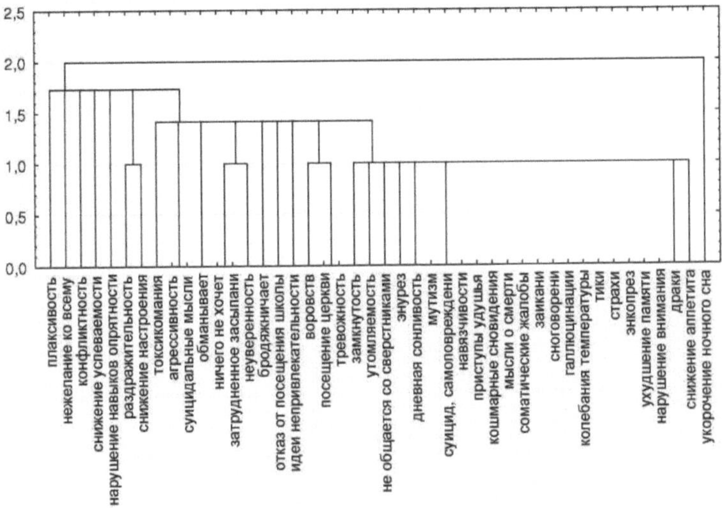

Figure 27. cluster analysis of mental state in mentally retarded children with a dysphoric type of clinical course of depressive disorder.

In all cases there was early alcoholization, smoking or drug use in the company of peers. Among girls of this group early sexual relations with aspiration to leave parents and to live with the sexual partners were encountered. Antidisciplinary behavior was characterized by a tendency to vagrancy, theft of tobacco products, alcohol or money, refusal to attend school, lack of reaction to parents' remarks. Because of the general intellectual underdevelopment, the antidisciplinary behavior as a whole was rather primitive, such children were to a greater degree slaves in the company of other children.

The clinical type of depression with mental regression in mental retardation revealed a prevalence of mental regression symptoms. This symptom complex is characteristic of all children with depression, but in the group of children with mental retardation its manifestations are the brightest. Appearance of so-called regressive (more precisely, pseudo-regressive) disorders, i.e. return to forms of behavior and skills, is characteristic of the younger age. Pseudo-regressive disorders in childhood depression are expressed in a temporary suspension of development when for weeks or even months, the addition of a vocabulary, acquisition of new motor functions, skills of self-care, more difficult forms of play stops (N.M. Iovchuk, A.A. Severny, 1998).

The unexpected occurrence of enuresis or encopresis in children with formed self-care skills prevailed in parents' complaints at hospitalization. There was a characteristic change of the child's behavior in the direction of childish forms: striving to play with children's toys, appearance of infantile intonations in speech, slovenliness in dressing and eating, refusal to use cutlery. Children did not communicate with peers, there was a decrease in school performance, they constantly cried, demanded to see them off in the street, answered questions inappropriately. They became overly compassionate: "sorry for the birds who are freezing in the street", "broken toys". Among older children, there was demonstrativeness, resentfulness, an excessive desire for cleanliness or refusal of hygienic procedures. Using the cluster analysis technique, we identified two main clusters of clinical manifestations (Fig. 28).

The regressive group manifested itself as enuresis or encopresis in children with formed neatness skills, puerile behavior: imitation in pronunciation of younger children, leering, loss of self-care skills, loss of acquired school knowledge. Children lost a sense of shame, could expose themselves or go to the toilet in front of strangers. Constantly demanded the presence of the mother or the tutor nearby, moved around, holding their hand. They refused to go to school by themselves and stayed home alone. They were afraid to communicate with surrounding adults and children. School progress was significantly lower: when studying according to the general education program, children refused to attend school, and when studying according to the remedial program, they lost the received knowledge. In some cases there was a loss of speech skills.

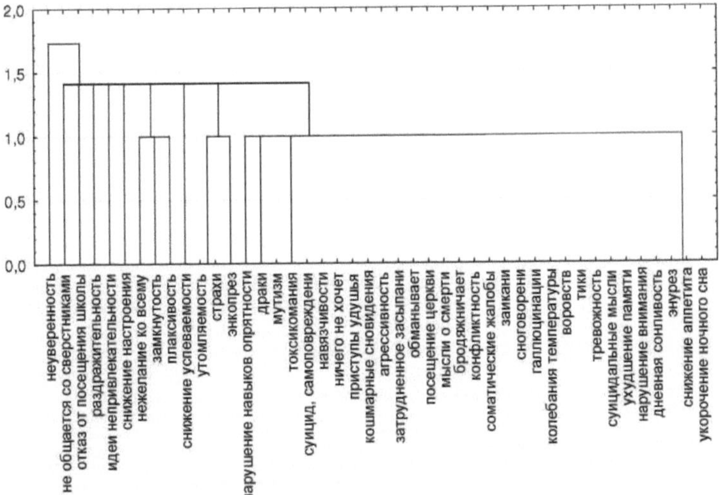

Figure 28. Cluster analysis of mental status in mentally retarded children with a regressive type of clinical course of depressive disorder.

The hypothymic group manifested itself in the form of adynamism, passivity, lowered mood, slowness, tearfulness, fearfulness, display of childhood fears (of Baba Yaga, "drubashka", doctors, policemen), the absence of positive emotional resonance was characteristic. As an illustration, here is a clinical observation of the patient.

Г. S., age 12. Admitted for the first time. Complains of tearfulness, attempts to draw attention to himself, tries to spend time near his mother, cries when parting, incontinence. Heredity was not psychopathologically burdened. He was brought up in a full family, the youngest child. There were three children in the family, the older children were healthy. Mother of 38 years old, secondary education, not working now. The father is 38 years old, education of 8 classes. The child was born from the 5th pregnancy, the third delivery at the age of 25 years old. Pregnancy went against the background of nephropathy of pregnant women, high blood pressure. The childbirth was on time, independent, weight at birth was 4600 grams. He screamed at once and was attached to the breast on the first day. Was discharged from the Maternity Hospital with the following condition: "A huge fetus, violation of cerebral circulation, grade I. Severe cerebral circulation disorder of the first degree. In the first year of life was observed by a neurologist with the diagnosis "Perinatal encephalopathy. He was once treated with nootropic agents. His psychomotor development was delayed: he began to sit up at 7 months, to walk at 1 year. He said his first words at the age of 3, developed his phraseology at the age of 5. Until one year of age he was a quiet, little-active child. In early childhood he was often ill with colds, vaccinated according to an individual schedule. At the age of 1.5, he had severe salmonellosis. He did not attend preschool, was brought up at home by his mother. He was an inactive child, reluctantly contacting the surrounding children, preferring family as his place of socialization. By character, his mother considered him quiet and shy. Neatness skills were formed at the age of 6.

He went to school at the age of 7 according to the program of a general education school. During studies in the first grade, he did not master the program; upon the recommendation of teachers, he underwent a medical-pedagogical commission. He was recommended to continue studying according to the program of a remedial school. Since the second grade up to the present time he has been studying in a remedial residential school. Since the beginning of remedial education he learned the program, did not stand out among his peers, and had friends in the class. On weekends parents took the child home. Now he was studying in the 4th grade. He did not have any traumas or surgeries under general anesthesia.

His condition changed within a month. He began to answer questions unilaterally, his grades dropped sharply, and he had trouble reproducing the learned knowledge. In class, he often talked in exaggerated childish speech. He refused to go with the class to group activities and to the canteen. In his free time, he tried to seclude himself, and did not answer the inquiries of the teachers. After some time, his mother noticed that the child was showing signs of fecal smut. At home, he spent all his time by his mother's side, "constantly holding her hand," refused to walk outside by himself, and asked to go to bed in his parents' bed. During the separation before the school week, he shouted, cried, would not let go of his mother, shouting: "You don't love me, you want to leave me here." At school, he stopped answering questions in class, refused to eat, did not wash his face, did not change his clothes, and had trouble falling asleep in the evening. We went to the psychiatrist on the teacher's recommendation.

Somatic condition: the condition is satisfactory, physique is correct, normosthenic. Skin, pharynx, visible mucous membranes of normal color, clean. Vesicular breathing, no rales on auscultation. The heart tones were clear and rhythmic. The abdomen was soft, painless, liver and spleen were not enlarged. Clinical and biochemical blood tests, general urinalysis without abnormal findings.

Neurological condition: eye slits are the same on both sides, pupils are rounded, reaction to light is preserved. Cranial innervation was not disturbed. Tendon reflexes in full volume, on both sides. The patient confidently performs coordination tests. No sensitivity disorders detected. EEG: irritation of the medial structures.

Mental state: correctly oriented in consciousness, place, time and personality. Mood background is lowered. Facial expression is sad, hypomimic. B conversation reluctantly. Often interrogates questions and answers one-sidedly. He speaks in an exaggeratedly childish voice. He is not at all interested in conversation and is burdensome to ask questions. He had difficulty giving his date of birth and does not remember his father's name and patronymic. He emphasized watching cartoons among his home occupations, but he did not remember the title, saying that "I always forget everything. He asked where his parents were, crying, "I want to go home to my mom. His knowledge and information were limited; he listed the seasons with help, but had difficulty naming the months, and did not name the distinctive features of the seasons. He failed to cope with the tasks of generalization and abstraction. He compared objects by secondary features. He constantly repeats, "I'm tired, can I go? He does not use the multiplication table in solving problems. He does not use help. Emotionally monotonous. Memory capacity is narrowed. The intellect is underdeveloped. Thinking of concrete-imaginative type, abstraction is poorly accessible.

During dynamic observation (for 33 days), he did not communicate with the children at first. He spent time alone, in his room. He did not participate in the general educational (visiting classes), game and therapeutic activities. He complained about tiredness, feeling unwell and "no mood. He ate under the control of the medical staff, "I don't want to. He had the phenomenon of fecal calamation. Constant control of hygienic measures was required. During treatment with Stimuloton 50 mg/day his condition improved. Mood was evened out, appetite and sleep improved. He began to communicate with younger children and play interests appeared. He attended the class, cope with the curriculum of the remedial school. Stool poisoning stopped on the third week of treatment.

Consultation of the psychologist: in the study of thinking activity the level of generalization, analysis, synthesis is decreased. Intellectual sphere with decrease. Abstraction is accessible partially. Thinking is sequential, concrete. Intelligence level below average (according to Wexler, verbal - 74, nonverbal - 68, general - 69). Appearance of depression on the Hamilton scale - 20 points, on the Kovacek school - 19 points.

Diagnosis: "Mild mental retardation, depressive behavior disorder.

Observation analysis: from early childhood, intellectual development was delayed, as a consequence of which a diagnosis of mild mental retardation was made. During the development there were manifestations of dysontogenesis (the stage of the first age crisis was characterized by delay of all components of normal ontogenesis, at the stage of the second age crisis there was separation of cognitive, affective, volitional and physical components with prevailing delay of intellectual development and reduced volitional activity) and social development disorders (the child did not attend preschool, had limited contacts with peers, was raised in a full family with prevailing type of education - "hypopedding"). At the moment of hospitalization, the change of the condition was associated with a depressive behavioral disorder manifested by regression of mental activity in the form of the appearance of encopresis, regressive childhood behavioral stereotypes (desire to constantly spend time with the mother, baby talk, isolation from the formed social environment, refusal of hygiene skills), decreased mood background, reduced appetite, disorders of night sleep.

3.4. Clinical features of the course of depressive mood disorders in children with organic mental disorders

A number of researches studied the clinical and psychopathological picture of depression within the limits of residual-organic neurosis-like conditions (V.M. Kozidubova, 1992; N.N. Kuzenkova, A.V. Chunikhina, 2004). The authors emphasize that the general clinical features of neurosis-like disorders are similar to psychogenic disorders of neurotic level in their phenomenological similarity, including relative poverty and monotone character of manifestations, more expressed organic coloring caused by close connection of neurosis-like disorders to psychorganic syndrome and residual organismic symptoms on cerebrasteanic background. B.N. Piven (1992) among typical signs of depressions of exogenous-organic nature, includes an asthenic patina, which is closely intertwined with depressive features and is most noticeable in the second half of the day. Patients reveal an exaggerated interpretation of various somatovegetative and psychopathological disorders, such as headaches, asthenization, dyssomnic phenomena, intellectual and mental difficulties. As the author notes, ODs develop against the background of residual-organic symptomatology, which not only accompanies them, but also precedes their occurrence, and also remains and intensifies in some cases after cessation of depression.

OD of this kind can develop at different time periods, and in the majority of patients they tend to recur periodically. L. S. Yusevich (1946), studying periodic mood disorders (dysphoria) in adolescent offenders with organic lesions of the brain, notes that this type of affective disorders is most common in psychopath-like states. In the clinical picture of "organic dysphoria" the most constant symptom is a wistful mood accompanied by anger, suspiciousness, hypochondriacal experiences, delusional ideas, headaches, a feeling of general weakness, brokenness. Depressive disorders are often registered among juvenile offenders with organic mental disorders. N.K. Demcheva and E.S. Natalevich (2000) conducted a study of psychogenically caused depressive disorders occurring in adolescents with organic mental disorders. The following features of psychogenic depressions on an organically impaired basis are allocated: high frequency of dysphoric and depressive-paranoid variants; polymorphism of a clinical picture and a protracted course of asthenodepressive conditions, sometimes taking the form of psychogenic development.

The atypical manifestations of depression are determined by the severity of the organic injuries suffered and the features of the pathological ground, including the age-related features of the maturation crisis. There is now evidence that fetal injuries, birth trauma, and other injuries that lead to the formation of a psychorganic syndrome have a higher risk of developing depression (Gillberg K., Hellgren L., 2004). Depressive-dysthymic neurosis-like states are disorders of the neurotic level of response arising in connection with cerebral disorders, which are caused by residual-organic brain disorders. Such conditions, according to V.S. Aleshko (1970), V.V. Kovalev (1995), have age differences. In children of preschool and younger school age, the low mood is combined with caprice, propensity to monotonous crying, quite often with vague fears. At high school age, a more expressed depressive affect with anxiety, hypochondriacal fears, irritability and dissatisfaction is noted. Adolescents occasionally have thoughts of their low worth and the uselessness of life. There are various vegetative disorders (hyperhidrosis, lack of appetite, vasoautonomic disorders), sleep disorders.

In a number of publications (Butorina N. E., Butorin G. G., 1999; Butorina N. E., 2004; Marcelli D., 1995) point out the close connection of depressive symptomatology to different forms of the psychoorganic syndrome. Thus V.M. Kozidubova (1992) allocates two variants of structure of depressive affect: the first - the combination of melancholy with anxiety, the second - with a prevalence of apathy. The author concludes, that the depressions of the posttraumatic genesis in children are characterized by relative simplicity of psychopathological structure, the picture of illness is complicated by the disorders included in structure of other symptoms, first of all cerebrasthenic.

Taking into account peculiarities of the clinical picture, 4 clinical variants of the course of depressive disorders in children with residual-organic CNS lesions have been allocated : dysphoric, hypochondriacal, regressive, simple.

The dysphoric clinical type of depression combined clinical types of depression with a prevalence of atypical malevolent affect, with dissatisfaction with others, irritability, short temper, along with ideational lethargy and complaints of a "bad", "angry" mood. A frequent reason for hospitalization of children was a suicide attempt (drug poisoning, vein dissection or attempts to throw oneself under a train) or the expression of suicidal threats or thoughts. In the remaining cases, parents complained about the children's resentfulness, dissatisfaction with others, and temper tantrums.

Behavior was oppositional and defiant: children damaged their and their parents' belongings, ran away from home, and wandered around. They reacted to educational measures with irritation, thoughts of unjust punishment, lack of appreciation by their parents ("no one understands me, they don't love me") or suicidal threats. They refused to go to school or broke discipline. School progress decreased, fatigue and a pessimistic outlook on life appeared. Children began to smoke, use alcoholic beverages, grouped with antisocial adolescents, and committed theft at home and in school. Attention deficit disorders and headaches appeared. In rare cases, children discontinued verbal contact with their parents altogether. Using the cluster analysis technique, we identified three main clusters of clinical manifestations (Fig. 29).

The <u>organoneuropathic group</u> included psychiatric syndromes caused by organic lesions of the CNS. The organic group included attention disorders with a tendency to exhaustion, deterioration of long-term and short-term memory, fatigability. The neurotic group was manifested by the child's anxiety, enuresis, encopresis, a shortened night's sleep, decreased appetite, lethargy, and somatic complaints. <u>The hypothymic group</u> united a lowered mood, verbalized by children as "angry", loss of former interests and urges. In general, the mood was gloomy, gloomy, joyless with absence of pleasure from any activity, dissatisfaction with themselves and others, hostility in a combination to reticence and tension.

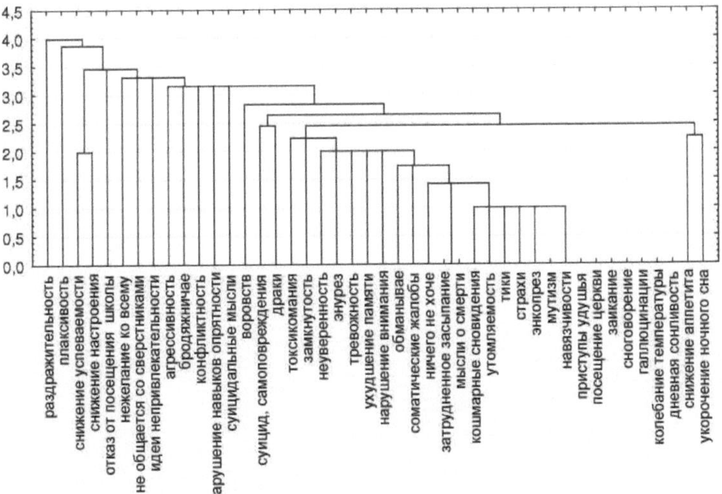

Fig. 29. cluster analysis of mental state in children with dysphoric type of clinical course of organic depressive disorder.

The dominant complaint of children was a feeling of resentment connected with the unfair attitude of others and abandonment.

Actively expressed ideas of their own unattractiveness. Episodes of crying occurred against a background of irritation. Expressed suicidal thoughts.

The psychopathic group was characterized by dissatisfaction with others, conflictedness, irascibility, irritability, outbursts of rage and aggression with a desire to destroy. Children stole money, spending it on sweets, computer games, cigarettes, alcohol. They stopped taking care of themselves (did not wash, did not change clothes). Blaming others for their condition, they preferred to spend time away from home, they roamed and fought. Learning disadaptation was characterized by the refusal to attend school, antidisciplinary, cynical behavior in school. Contact with peers and former friends was broken, the children aspired to join antisocial groups. They committed suicide attempts or injured themselves. To illustrate, we will cite a clinical observation of a patient.

Observat
ion 5

P. A., 12 years old. Comes in for the first time. Complaints on admission: refusal to go to school, irritability, fits of anger, lowered mood. Heredity was not psychopathologically burdened. Mother was 34 years old, higher education, worked as an engineer. Father, 37 years old, secondary technical education, works as a foreman. The elder sister was 15 years old and was not in poor health. The child was born from the fourth pregnancy, which had toxemia in the first half of the pregnancy and anemia in the second half. Prior to this pregnancy, she had one physiological delivery and two medical abortions. Second term delivery, fetal weight at birth was 3900 grams. The diagnosis of perinatal encephalopathy, hematomas was made during delivery. On the third day of life he was transferred to the department of pathology of newborns with the diagnosis: "Perinatal encephalopathy, cerebral edema". For 6 days he stayed in the intensive care unit, after which he was transferred to the neonatology department and discharged two weeks later.

In the first year of his life, he was not observed by a neurologist and received no treatment. He grew up calm, had no complaints about his behavior or health. Motor development according to his age: he held his head at 2 months, sat up at 6 months, walked at 10 months. The delay in mental development also was not noted: the first words till one year of age, the phrase speech by two years old. At the age of 2 1/2, there was a closed head injury, obtained while playing with his sister. Hit his head on the radiator, loss of consciousness was noted, was hospitalized in the hospital, where he was treated for 7 days with the diagnosis of brain contusion. At the age of 3.5, there was a repeated CTSD - he slipped in the bathroom, loss of consciousness, nausea, vomiting were also noted. He was hospitalized for 3 weeks with the diagnosis "concussion of brain". After that, he became irritable, often cried and was restless. From the diseases he had: frequent acute respiratory infections. Supervised by gastroenterologist for dolichosygmia. At the age of 11, under general anesthesia he had a surgery for inguinal hernia. He did not attend preschool, but attended it at his parents' request. Had little contact with his peers. He went to school at 7, mastered the program, communicated little with children. From school features: he had good academic abilities, but was passive and got tired quickly during lessons.
He is withdrawn by character, often immersed in his own thoughts, but he complies with all requirements of the teachers. Relationships with classmates are uneven, he prefers to be alone and keeps away from children. Adaptation in a new team is hard, he does not show initiative in communication.

He first consulted a psychiatrist when he was 8 years old because he was irritable, aggressive toward relatives, did not react to comments, expressed thoughts about not wanting to live, at school he fought with classmates, could swear at the teacher during a lesson, could not sit through a lesson. During his examination by the psychiatrist, he did not talk to the doctor and did not comply with his requests. He was diagnosed with the following condition: "Respiratory-organic CNS lesion, psychopathic-like syndrome. He was treated with nootropics and behavior correctors (Sonapax). During the course of treatment, his condition slightly improved. The child's condition changed at the age of 3 months. He refused to go to school, went to classes, but did not attend class. He often repeated that he was tired, got tired of school, expressed thoughts about not wanting to live, spoke about "the absence of vital energy. At school, he was inactive and exhausted, and his school performance dropped drastically. By the decision of the local psychiatrist, he was transferred to home schooling. However, there was no improvement in his condition. He continued to actively express thoughts about not wanting to live, and was irritable. There were episodes during which he threatened to stab himself or close relatives. For a month, he spent most of his time away from home, and his mother noticed that he smelled like alcohol and tobacco. He had little contact with his parents, and in response to comments, he threatened suicide. His mood was constantly lowered with irritation. He was admitted at his parents' request and on the referral of the local psychiatrist.

Somatic condition: physique is correct, normosthenic. The skin was clean, of normal color, and the pharynx was calm. Breathing was vesicular, no rales on auscultation. The heart tones were clear and rhythmic. The abdomen was soft and painless. The liver and spleen were not enlarged. Physiological excretion was normal. Clinical and biochemical blood tests, general urinalysis without abnormal findings.

Neurological condition: eye slits are the same on both sides, pupils are rounded, reaction to light is preserved. Cranial innervation is not impaired. Static and coordination were not disturbed. No sensitivity disorders were revealed. EEG: moderate diffuse changes of bioelectrical processes of dysrhythmic nature with predominance of polymorphic and slow-wave theta-band activity in the recording. No focal and interhemispheric asymmetry was detected. No epi-activity was detected. ECHOES: no evidence of displacement of midline brain structures.

Mental state: Reluctant to come into contact, wary. He is oriented correctly. Attention is attracted, but is quickly exhausted in the process of conversation. The stock of general domestic and school knowledge is at the lower limit of the age norm. He complains about frequent headaches on his own. He falls asleep poorly, as "different thoughts" come into his head before he goes to sleep about how he is going to deal with his abusers. He has a poor appetite - "sometimes I don't want to eat at all. He considers his mood bad for 3-4 months, "several months ago, I didn't want to live; now I don't want to live either, I'm bored with everything, I'm bored, I have no friends. He is indifferent to conversation, a little lethargic. Emotionally unstable, mood background is lowered. Memory, intellect without major defects. Thinking at a somewhat slower pace, abstraction available.

In the course of dynamic observation (for 43 days), at first, his mood remained lowered in the ward, he adapted poorly, remained isolated, did not communicate with children. Periodic episodes of dysphoria with aggression directed at children or medical staff. After treatment with Stimuloton 25 mg/day, Cortexin and participation in psychotherapy group, his mood improved, he became more sociable, played with children willingly, attended the class, mastered the curriculum. He became friendly at home, and his sleep and appetite improved.

Consultation of the psychologist: fatigability and exhaustion of attention of the organic type, peculiarities of the emotional-volitional sphere (decreased background of mood, emotional lability). Hamilton scale - 23 points, Kovacek scale - 11 points before treatment, Dahl school: 7-8 years.

Diagnosis: "Organic personality disorder with affective disorders. Current depressive episode.

Surveillance analysis: born from the 4th pregnancy, with PEP, cerebral edema. Did not receive adequate treatment in the first year of life. Subsequently, he had two recurrent CTS and surgery under general anesthesia. Impaired social development (did not attend preschool, had difficulty finding contacts with his peers, pathological type of upbringing "inconsistent type of upbringing" was noted). At present, a repeated depressive episode, the first one at the age of 8 years was not diagnosed. The condition is defined by the decreased mood with aggressive and autoaggressive actions, vegetative disturbances (sleep and appetite), dysphoric inclusions (occasional use of alcohol and tobacco smoking, aggression toward relatives and peers). A current depressive episode (dysphoric clinical type) in a patient with an organic personality disorder was identified.

The *hypochondriacal clinical type* of depression combined depression with a prevalence of symptoms of somatic malaise. Children in this group were repeatedly examined by general somatic specialists and received general strengthening treatment without any effect. Pointing to the modification of children's condition, parents noted a large number of somatic complaints of asthenic and hypochondriacal content without clear organ localization. All children had appetite disorders until refusal to eat, sleep in the form of difficulties in falling asleep, interruptions, and superficiality of sleep. Children were withdrawn from their worries, isolated from others, reluctant to go to school or were withdrawn completely due to poor well-being. Episodes of general malaise were interrupted by outbursts of irritability with tears, expressing thoughts of death. Children lost interest in the formerly interesting activities or completely lost interest in life, and in order to attract attention, they spoiled things. Using the clustering technique, we identified two main clusters of clinical manifestations (Fig. 30).

The <u>asthenoid hypochondriac group</u> included complaints of an asthenic somatic state change (weakness, lethargy, fatigue, headaches, unpleasant bodily sensations, intolerance of academic workload), reduction and perversion of eating behavior, appearance of fears of a possible severe somatic disease ("I have cancer, AIDS, I will die soon"). Sleep disorders in the form of shortening, difficulties in falling asleep, nightmares, lack of a sense of sleep, general anxiety, hyperesthesia to bright light or sound were noted. Manifestations of the asthenic symptom complex prevailed in the first half of the day in the form of weakness, slowness, lethargy and boredom. In the evening, tearfulness, motor restlessness and irritability increased.

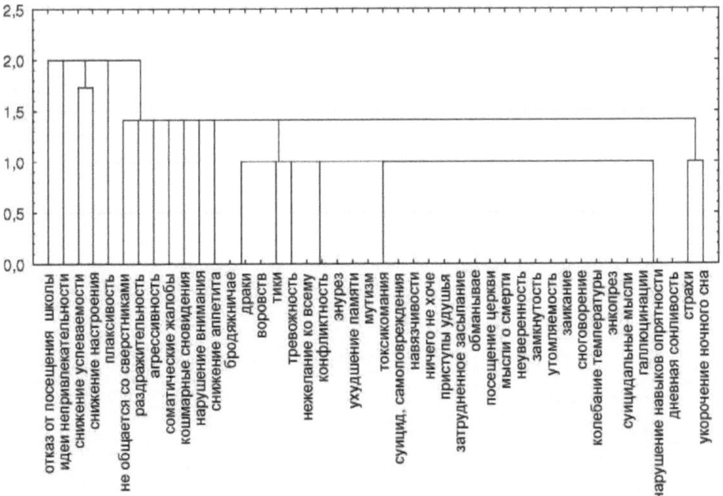

Figure 30. Cluster analysis of mental status in children with hypochondriacal type of clinical course of organic depressive disorder.

The hypothymic-organic group combined lowered mood in the form of boredom, dissatisfaction, and depression. Children became tearful, tried to draw attention to themselves, expressing ideas of their unattractiveness. School disadaptation was connected not only with the general depressive background, but also with exhaustion of attention, an uneven rate of mental performance, stiffness of thinking.

The clinical type of depression with mental regression combined depression with the occurrence of pseudoregressive disorders. Often patients with these complaints consulted various specialists - neurologists, psychologists and psychiatrists, where they received treatment for neurosis-like symptoms (fears, enuresis, encopresis). However, the medical treatment received did not lead to a reduction of the symptomatology. At the hospitalization stage, parents complained about mental changes of neurotic character, which were typical for young children. The complaints of the emergence of fears of infantile contents prevailed: own death and death of parents, fear of nonexistent events or objects, fear of animals not available in our region.

Children's behavior changed according to these fears: they tried to spend time at home, together with parents, they were suspicious of others. They reacted negatively to attempts of dissuasion with elements of irritation, ending in tears, and positive emotional events and activities did not cause them an emotional response. Children had enuresis or encopresis. Parents noticed some infantilism in the children's statements and behavior. School maladaptation with difficulties in mastering the school curriculum appeared. Using the cluster analysis technique, we identified two main clusters of clinical manifestations (Fig. 31).

The regressive-neurotic group was characterized by the occurrence of neurotic symptomatology (fears, neatness, anxiety, compulsive movements), which had a primitive-infantile character. Children became suggestible - after the tragic events in Beslan, the fear of death at school. Troubles arising in the families of friends and the immediate neighborhood, were transferred to the own family (divorce, parents' illnesses), and viewing films formed a fear of transferring the events of the film to real life ("I can be eaten by a crocodile"). Sleep disorders in the form of difficulty falling asleep and nightmares appeared. Episodes of crying were consistently accompanied by questions: "Will there be no war?", "I won't die?

The hypotymic-organic group was manifested by an undifferentiated lowered mood with pronounced manifestations of ideational lethargy. Children restricted themselves in contacts, often complained of weariness. They expressed naive occasional ideas of self-blaming and self-deprecation: "I torture my mom, I do not eat porridge," "I am bad, I cannot ride a bicycle," and their subject matter was limited to family and school problems.

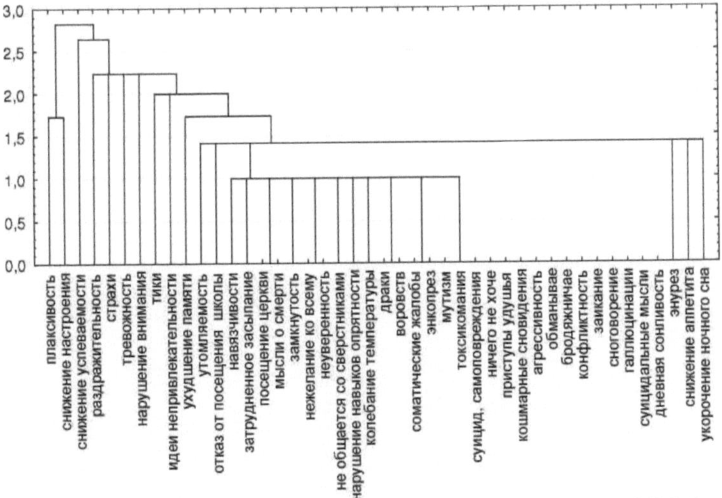

Figure 31. Cluster analysis of mental status in children with a regressive type of clinical course of organic depressive disorder.

The asthenic component of psychoorganic origin was characterized by fatigability, impaired attention, a decrease in the rate of mental performance with a fading phenomenon. At school, children had difficulty reproducing the received knowledge, often refused to answer verbally, complaining of "no thoughts in the head: "I do not remember anything", "I am tired". B in the moment of a psychologically traumatic situation, they would switch to exaggeratedly childish speech.

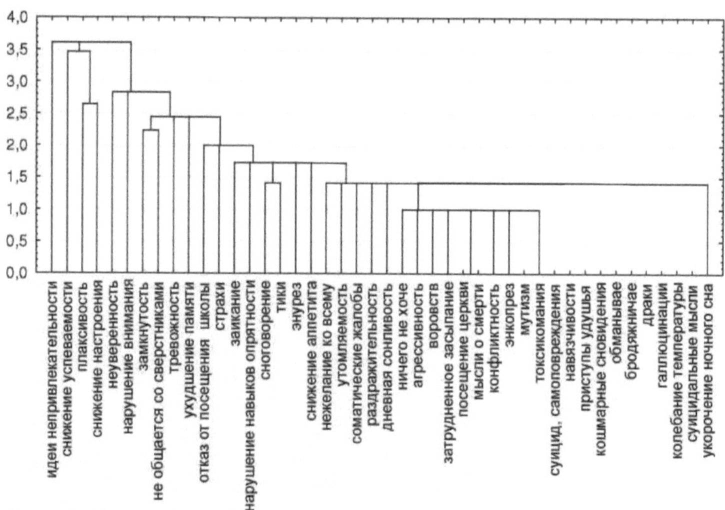

Figure 32. Cluster analysis of mental status in children with a simple type of clinical course of organic depressive disorder.

The *simple clinical type* of depressive disorder combined depression with little differentiated lowered mood, predominance of sadness and grief, pessimistic assessment of the present and future, and lowered self-esteem. At hospitalization, parents complained about general weakness, fatigability, passivity, lack of interest in life, and a lowered mood. Children had a sharp drop in their academic performance, and a negative attitude toward school study was formed. Children became tearful, reluctant to tell their parents about their anxiety. A decrease in motor activity was noted, and previously active children preferred to spend time "lying on the sofa," did not communicate with friends, ceased to be engaged in the activities which had previously interested them. Using the clustering technique, two main clusters of clinical manifestations were identified (Fig. 32).

The hypotymic group was characterized by a decrease in mood with ideas of general unattractiveness or insolvency, insecurity, and tearfulness. There was a disappearance of positive emotional reactions or general animation when meeting acquaintances. Children became non-smiling, preferred to spend time alone, complained of boredom, physical malaise or fatigue. They refused to read, watch TV programs. Their ability to study was sharply decreased; children either passively attended school or completely refused to study without explaining the reasons ("I can't," "I don't want," "I won't study").

The vegetative-organic group was characterized by disturbance of the sleep-wake regime in the form of a shortening of night sleep, difficulties in falling asleep, nightmares and daytime sleepiness. There was an eating disorder, decreased appetite. During the day, if there were no reminders from parents, children refused to eat at all, and if parents insisted, they ate selectively, in small portions (only sweet or their favorite food). They periodically complained of palpitations, dizziness, headaches or unpleasant bodily sensations in various parts of the body. The organic component of depression mimicked character pathology and was characterized by episodic outbursts of irritability, conflict or theft. Children stole money from parents, buying sweets for classmates, or took their own or parents' things out of the house and gave them to others.

Thus, a cluster analysis of syndromic symptoms showed that in children with depression on the background of schizophrenia, the hypochondriacal type was manifested by somatohypothymic, hallucinatory-depressed and apatoabolic clinical manifestations. The magyphrenic clinical type revealed a symptom complex of
vegetati
ve-confessional, apathetic, and hypothymic disorders. The autoaggressive clinical type of depression included clinical symptoms, which were defined by hypothymic, psychopathic-like and autoaggressive manifestations. The dysphoric type in schizophrenic depression was characterized by psychopath-like manifestations. The simple clinical type of depression was represented by ideational disorders and hypothymic manifestations. The anxious-phobic clinical type was characterized by hypothymic and neurotic manifestations. In children with neurotic depression, the dysphoric clinical type was characterized by asthenoneurotic, psychopathic-like, and hypothymic-dysphoric disorders,

clinically framed by vegetative and hypothymic-hypothymic manifestations. Anxiety-phobic type of depression was manifested by dysphoric, hypotimic-anxious, and hypotimic-phobic symptoms. The simple clinical type of depression was characterized by vegetative-dysphoric and hypothymic components. The simple type, manifested by hypothymic and vegetative manifestations, was recorded for depression on the background of mental retardation. The dysphoric type was outlined by hypothymic symptomatology and psychopathic disorders. The regressive type was characterized by a regressive and hypothymic symptom complex.

In organic depressive disorders, the dysphoric type was defined by organoneuropathic, hypothymic and psychopath-like symptoms. The hypochondriac type was characterized by asthenoipochondriacal and hypotymic-organic symptomocomplexes. Clinical type with regression of mental development was manifested by symptoms of regressive-neurotic and hypotymic-organic character. The simple clinical type was defined by hypotymic and vegetative-organic symptoms.

3.5. Age-related pathomorphosis of the depressive syndrome in the process of personality formation

Studying the manifestation of depressive symptoms in children, the problem of considering the child not as a "static element" of the formed adult personality, but as a "continuously developing" object, undergoing changes in the process of physiological and psychological growing up is actualized. At the same time, the clinical manifestations of DP are not static either and undergo development in the course of the child's ontogenesis. F. Antropov (2001), studying the age-specific features of MD in children, has revealed some features of depression at various age stages. Thus, features of depression in the first year of life of the child are weak intensity, incompleteness and transience of symptoms. A newborn infant in the first year of life reacts to adverse influences not only by crying, whimpering, crying, moodiness, anxiety, lethargy, apathy, decreased motor activity, but also by sleep disorders such as a shortening or interruption of sleep, decreased appetite and regurgitation, changes in skin color and thermoregulation. If DN is more severe, crying is prolonged, prolonged insomnia with short sleep, refusal to breastfeed, poor weight gain and stunted growth. While anxious, restless, crying children have relatively differentiated facial expressions and during periods of positive stimuli, other children with a more pronounced decrease in emotional tone do not respond to entertaining activities, and they are characterized by sullen concentration. The vegetative component of depression manifests itself in the form of allergic reactions, disorders of the gastrointestinal tract, thermoregulation.

During the period from 1 to 4 years of age, clinical manifestations of depression undergo changes because this period of childhood is characterized by active cognition of the environment, expansion of the range of interests and emotional reactions to what is going on. The clinic of depression is characterized by lowered mood outside of conflict situations and is manifested by a decrease in positive emotions in facial expressions or prevalence of negative emotions. Children limit social contacts, become sad, their reasoning is related to unpleasant moments in their lives, complain of boredom, sadness, and are often offended. They react negatively to placement in children's institutions, and are anxious about parental delays. Sleep disorders appear in the form of late falling asleep, restlessness at night or waking up out of fear. Appetite is reduced, body weight is insufficient, with long-term depressive disorders there is a growth retardation.

The clinic of depression in preschool children (5-6 years old) is defined by the awakening of self-awareness, the child does not tolerate injustice, restrictions of activity. In this connection, the lowered mood of the child is characterized not only by sadness, but also acquires a shade of dissatisfaction, conflictedness and aggression. At younger school age (7-9 years old), depressions become more delineated and are characterized by greater dependence on the external situation. Dullness is often associated with school attendance, communication with classmates and teachers. Children experience boredom both in and out of lessons; they explain their lack of productivity by a bad mood or unwillingness to do anything; they often reveal a tendency to distract themselves somehow, to improve their condition by playing games, eating sweets, or skipping lessons. Productivity in classes suffers due to impaired attention, memory, concentration, and asthenia. Hypothymia is characterized as sadness, melancholy, boredom, sadness. The spectrum of somatic disorders here is much wider than in the case of depression at younger ages. At the pre-adolescent age (10-11 years old), MDs manifest themselves more definitely, and children have a more delicate sense of their emotional state and can characterize it more definitely. Complaints concern not only boredom and despondency, but also displeasure and depression. Affective displays become relatively stable and more pronounced. In adolescent patients (12-

17 years old) clinical manifestations become more pronounced and complex, approaching those of adults.

Studying features of depressive disorders in children, three age periods were singled out to determine the age-specific pathomorphosis of depressive symptoms: elementary school age (6-8 years), school age (9-11 years), and pre-adolescence (12-14 years). Having carried out the process of clusterization of symptoms of depression in these age groups, we managed to identify the main groups of clinical manifestations of hypothymic disorders, characteristic for a certain age period. The clinic of depressive symptoms in the younger school age is defined to a greater degree by the crisis of the seventh year of life associated with transition of the child from preschool to school age and with a fundamental change of the child's position in society, i.e. with a change of the social situation of development (Elkonin D.B., 1978).

As research shows, the so-called "crisis of 7 years" begins already at age 6 (Elkonin D.B., Wenger A.L., 1988). And the child for the first time has socially significant obligations which fulfillment is estimated not only by close adults, but also by a representative of society - the teacher. The child's psychological "appropriation" of the new social status is reflected in the rejection of "preschool" orientations and in the formation of an internal position of the schoolboy.

Relationships with family members and friends are the most significant for the preschooler.

Such relations are built as direct, defined by love, sympathies or antipathies of the child, being based on the experience of communication with the given concrete people. In contrast, for the younger schoolboy the relations not defined by direct interpersonal contacts are of paramount importance (Shevchenko Y. S., Venger A. L., 2006).

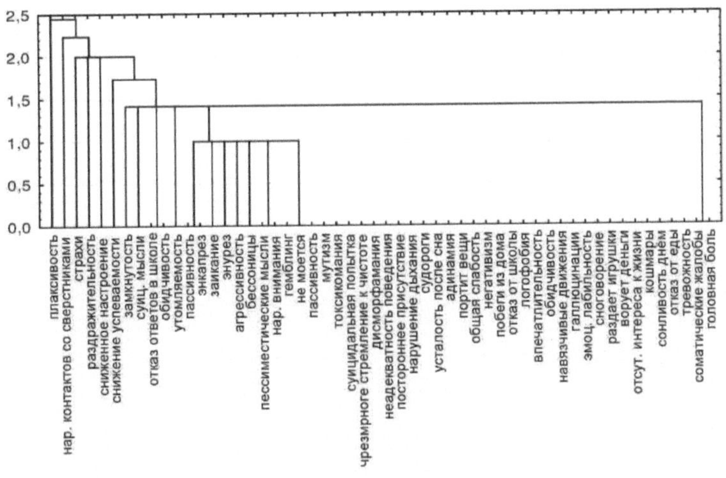

Figure 33. Cluster analysis of clinical manifestations of depressive disorders in children of primary school age.

Depressive manifestations in younger school age were characterized by an undifferentiated lowered mood with masking of hypothymic symptomatology by tearfulness, resentfulness, passivity, and violation of personal hygiene skills (Fig. 33).

Children were reluctant to communicate with other children, had a negative attitude toward the beginning of school, learned program material with difficulty, often caused a negative attitude towards them by their appearance and behavior of other children. Some children defiantly refused to go to school, predicting "trouble. Other children, while having a calm attitude toward learning, quickly became exhausted during the first lessons and lost interest in learning. Often in these children an anxious component was noted in the form of fears, which had the character of both physiological childhood and tended to be somewhat globalized, covering familiar areas of life (family, school) for the child.

The anxious component was accompanied by irritability of the child, connected with demands in dissuasion of his fears. The vegetative component of depression was manifested by an increase in the number of somatic complaints of asthenic content, without clear organ localization, sleep disorders with difficulty falling asleep, scary dreams, insufficient feeling of rest in the morning. Depressive disorders were accompanied by a neurosis-like component in the form of enuresis, encopresis and stuttering. The clinical manifestations of depressive disorders fall into three main groups: 1) impaired social functioning of the child; 2) anxious-hypothymic manifestations; and 3) asthenoneurotic manifestations.

The clinic of DN in school-age children was determined to a greater extent by the formed position of the schoolboy. The child was adapting in a new social position, acquiring an orientation to a wide social environment. The social significance of learning activity was determined by consistent, systematic training of the child. The position of the pupil in learning activities becomes meaningful - the child is aware of his/her role in learning activities. The child's social environment and relations in all existing systems - "child - family", "child - teachers", "child - children" (Shevchenko Y. S., Venger A. L., 2006) are fully formed. Owing to this short-term psychological stability, depressive manifestations in school-age children are characterized by less polymorphism of clinical manifestations, but by a more bright selection of the classical depressive triad.

The hypothymic symptomatology detected in the majority of patients was connected not only with the brightness of clinical manifestations, but also with the ability of children of the given age to designate their lowered mood as sad,

sad, bad. Reduced mood was accompanied by tearfulness,   pessimism,
resentfulness, passivity,
children became irritable, tearful, refused to answer at school, left lessons, spent time in the company of older or younger children. The dysphoric component alternated with hypothymic symptomatology; children often repented of their actions, cried, asked for forgiveness. In general, dysphoric displays were short-lived, had an incomplete character and were manifested by oppositional defiant acts (stealing money, spoiling things, personal unkemptness).

Apathetic symptomatology was defined by the violation of contacts with peers, reticence, general adynamy, absence of interest in life. Children could hardly cope with program material, required a considerable amount of time to master new material, and parents noticed a pronounced decrease in their children's school performance. The vegetative component of depression was represented by extensive somatic symptoms of the general vegetative profile, having a clear organ projection (gastrointestinal tract: abdominal pain, dyspepsia; respiratory system: respiratory disorders, a feeling of suffocation). Neurotic symptomatology was defined by the presence of enuresis, encopresis, stuttering.

Clinical manifestations of depression were subdivided into 1) hypothymic manifestations; 2) dysphoric disorders; and 3) neurotic manifestations of the obscheurotic and hypochondriacal profiles (Fig. 34).

The clinical picture of depressive displays in children of pre-adolescence (12-14 years) is defined by initial displays of a crisis of adolescence (Elkonin, D.B., 1978). The social situation of development at this age is being reconstructed, and the degree of independence increases. In pre-adolescence age, in spite of the fact that school training proceeds, educational activity recedes into the background. The leading activity becomes construction of a system of new social relations, the child is not satisfied with his or her place in the system of relations which adults present to him or her, he or she tries to independently

He or she tries to independently choose the activity he or she is ready to perform. In relations with adults, the child strives for full equality.

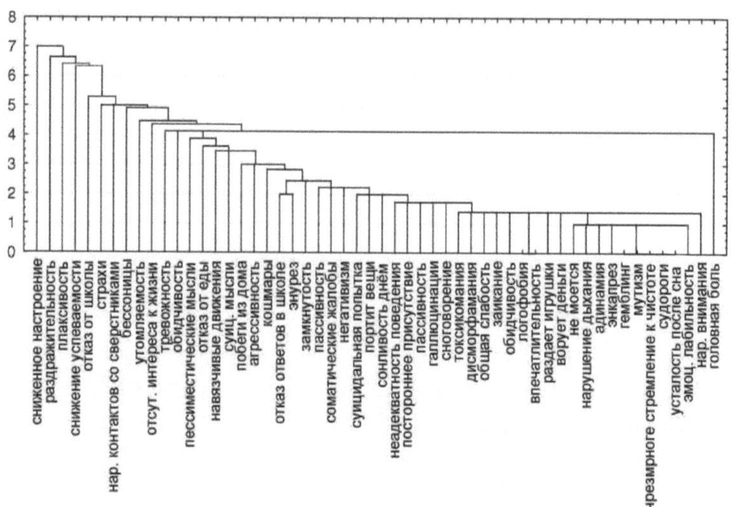

Figure 34. Cluster analysis of clinical manifestations of depressive disorders in school-age children.

The adult loses the function of the teacher and gets the function of the senior partner to be estimated (Shevchenko Y. S., Venger A. L., 2006). Functioning of the child at this stage is represented by various kinds of social interaction and is embodied not only in interpersonal communication with peers (Elkoni D.B., 1989), in socially useful activity (Feldstein D.I., 1999), but also in negativism, rudeness.

The clinical picture of depressive manifestations in pre-adolescent children is more definite, expressed and complex than in the previous age periods. At this age, children are able to differentiate their mood as lowered, often complaining of sadness, despondency, a feeling of boredom. They directly relate all of these feelings to a lowered mood (Fig. 35). However, the obviously lowered mood is combined with pronounced negativism of the child. In connection with the beginning of the teenage crisis, the child's relations with society become not so much social, more likely even antisocial, and learning activity ceases to be leading. Children resolutely refuse to go to school, skip classes, clash with teachers at school, aspire to communicate with groups of asocial teenagers.

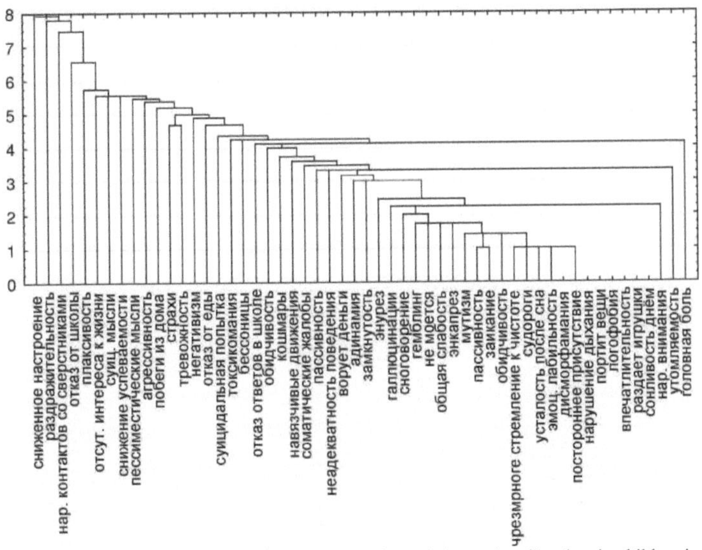

Figure 35. Cluster analysis of clinical manifestations of depressive disorders in children in pre-adolescence.

Even if the child did well at school before the onset of depression, later, it is not uncommon to find difficulty in learning along with the appearance of depressive symptoms. The ideational component of depression is manifested in the form of slowness of thinking, compulsive recollections of the unpleasant experiences.

Asocial behavior is determined not only by the beginning of the pubertal crisis, but also by the appearance of depressive symptoms. At the same time, the depressive symptomatology colors the dysphoric symptomatology with the desire to do harm not only to others, but also to themselves: children begin to actively express suicidal thoughts or commit suicide attempts, alcoholic or substance abuse excesses occur (substance abuse by volatile carbons or tobacco smoking).

Asthenic symptomatology is manifested by a decrease in motor activity and productivity of activity, intensifying in the afternoon, and children begin to require an afternoon rest.

The neurotic symptomatology becomes rather bright and is defined by the anxious component and the appearance of wistful affect. Unlike other age groups, anxiety is rarely accompanied by a phobic component, but is globalized, covering all habitual areas of the child's activity, including the child's personal health. This feature is connected with ontogenesis of the psychological development of the child and the self-consciousness being formed at this age stage. The somatic components of depressive disorders are rather diverse and are manifested by extensive vegetovisceral disorders of the skin, digestive, respiratory, motor and other organs and systems, as well as algic manifestations, along with which disorders of the cardiovascular, endocrine systems and eating behavior are revealed. At the same time, the dependence of somatovegetative disorders on the severity of depression is always noted. Thus, clinical manifestations of depression in this age group are defined by: 1) depressive-dysfunctional, 2) anxious-distressing, and 3) somatoalgic manifestations.

Comparing the clinical manifestations of DN in children in the selected age groups, it was shown that DN in the elementary school age are characterized by autoaggressive clinical forms (11.1%) of the course. However, simple (27.8%) and dysphoric (27.8%) forms were more common in the clinical manifestations of DN (Table 2).

In children of school age, simple (35.4%), hypochondriac (13.8%), anxious-phobic (14.6%) and regressive (11.5%) clinical forms of the course of depressive disorders were the most common. In the clinical picture of depression at this age, simple (35.4 %) and dysphoric (22.3 %) forms prevailed. At the pre-adolescent age there was an increase of dysphoric (37.4 %) and magiphrenic (5.7 %) clinical types of the course of depression. In general, dysphoric (37.4%), simple (24.9%) and anxiety-phobic (12.9%) clinical forms are more common at this age.

Table 2

Distribution of clinical types of the course of depressive disorders in children depending on age periods

Clinical types of depression	6-8 years old		Years 9-11		12-14 years old	
	abs.	%	abs.	%	abs.	%
Dysphoric	5	27,8	29	22,3	72	37,4
Hypochondriac	2	11,1	18	13,8	19	9,8
Simple	5	27,8	46	35,4	48	24,9
Anxiety-phobic	1	5,55	19	14,6	25	12,9
Autoaggressive	2	11,1	1	0,8	6	3,1
Magifrenic	1	5,55	2	1,6	11	5,7
Regressive	2	11,1	15	11,5	11	6,2
Total	18	5,3	130	38,1	193	56,6

Thus, it has been found that the clinical course of depressive disorders in children depends on the age period of occurrence. At younger school age, during the "crisis of 7 years", there was a disturbance of social functioning of the child with anxious-hypothymic and asthenoneurotic manifestations. Among clinical forms, both simple (27.8%) and dysphoric (27.8%) were equally common. As the child grew older, during school age, the polymorphism of clinical depressive manifestations increased, with the classical depressive triad being more prominent.

The clinical picture was defined by hypothymic, neurotic manifestations of the obscheurotic and hypochondriacal profile, and dysphoric disorders. Among clinical forms, there was an increase in simple (35.4%) and a decrease in dysphoric (22.3%). In pre-adolescence, the clinical picture of depressive manifestations in children was more definite, pronounced and complex than in previous age periods, masked by manifestations of the negative stage of the adolescent pubertal crisis, defined by depressive-dysphoric, anxious-dysphoric and somatoalgic manifestations. In the clinical course, the number of dysphoric (37.4%) clinical forms increased and the number of simple forms decreased (24.9%).

CONCLUSION.

Children's mental health determines the health of the nation in the future and occupies one of the leading places in the prevention of mental health pathology worldwide, defining one of the most urgent tasks of Russian psychiatry (V.Y. Semke, 2004). In recent decades, there has been an increase in mental disorders in all countries of the world, and Russia in particular. To a greater extent, it concerns adolescents and children. A number of authors emphasize a major role in the emergence of an increase in childhood mental disorders of the crisis situation which developed in Russia in the mid-1990s (Dmitrieva, T. B., 2001). Epidemiological research conducted by various authors in different regions of Russia indicate an increase in non-psychotic mental disorders, mental retardation and exogenous-organic disorders (Bryzgin M.B., 1995; Tazlova R.S., 1998; Sukhotina N.K., 2000; Kuzenkova N.N., Treshutin V. A., 2002; Levina I. L., 2003; Shmakova O. П., 2004). Thus, in 1991, the incidence of mental disorders among children was 425.1 per 100,000 of the population, and in 2003, it rose to 639.1. The indicators of morbidity also increased, 2,344.8 in 1991 and 3,249.0 in 2001, respectively. The greatest increase in these indicators was noted in the Urals and Siberian regions (Goskomstat of the Russian Federation, 1997).

The methodological basis for the study of childhood mental disorders should be the systems approach as the most adequate tool in modern scientific research. Methods of the system analysis are widely used for the solution of many theoretical and applied problems. The historical preconditions and philosophical foundations of the system approach in works by B.G. Ananyev (1969), B.F. Lomov (1975), V.P. Kuzmin (1982) have been studied rather completely. Currently, the systems approach is being applied more and more widely in psychiatry, and experience is being accumulated in constructing systemic descriptions of objects of research.

The need for a systems approach is due to the enlargement and complication of the studied systems, the needs of managing large systems and the integration of knowledge. The term "systems approach" covers a group of methods by which a real object is described as a set of interacting components. The system approach allows us to determine the generality of mental phenomena with other phenomena of objective reality. As a result of application of the system approach it is possible to receive system descriptions of the complex phenomena of objective reality (Ganzen V. A., 1984).

In this paper, we have considered the child-environment system as a dynamic one, since the existence, functioning and development of the child is determined not only by the genetic program, but also by social influence. Realization of social influence is made possible through the interaction of the individual with the environment and purposeful influence on it. In order to build a systemic description, the object of the systemic model, in accordance with the objectives of the study, was a child with a depressive mood disorder. The use of this approach has allowed to develop a clinical typology of depressive disorders and to present a connection between the psychopathological structure of the depressive syndrome and nosological affiliation. The types of "pathological ground" or dysontogenesis identified in children with depression (Gurieva V.A., 2001) allow to improve early diagnosis of depressive disorders in childhood and to develop specialized preventive programs.

Preventive   (preventive)   direction is the fundamental principle of mental health care for children. WHO experts predict a shift in the strategy and tactics of modern medicine toward the promotion and development of mental health. The concept of mental health care for children should be based on the creation of practical models of "fair preventive-oriented health services, including the promotion of healthy lifestyles, widespread disease prevention, control of risk factors and the provision of adequate primary care" (Semke V.Y., 1999; Gutkevich E.V., Semke V.Y., 2004). In recent years, prerequisites for formation of the idea of preventive psychiatry have been created, which considers the problem of strengthening and saving of mental health of children through a system of correcting pathogenic and strengthening sanogenic mechanisms of external and internal spheres, with the ultimate goal to restore a healthy way of life (V.Y. Semke, 1995, 1999, 2002, 2004).

Further progress in the field of thorough study and promotion of mental health is possible only through the systematic use of new methodological approaches, among which the most promising should be recognized *the clinical and epidemiological* (which allows to fully assess the "magnitude of problems" of socio-hygienic situation in a particular region), *clinical and dynamic* (covering different "poles" and "transitions" in the continuum "health - illness") and *rehabilitative* ("closing" the results of the previous two approaches and solving problems of both prevention and complex therapy). The problem of improving mental health indicators cannot be solved outside of a multidisciplinary study of the psychohygienic foundations of prevention and early diagnosis of neuropsychiatric disorders. Creation on the basis of existing and newly organized multilevel systems of human health protection (including the problem of "healthy health") with separate stages of implementation of specific results allows to obtain direct scientific and practical effect, and their combination will provide a steady tendency of growth of indicators of both individual and public health.

LITERATURE

1 . Avdeeva, N. N. Psychology of your baby / N. N. Avdeeva, S. Meshcheryakova, V. G. Razhnikova. - M. : AST, 1996.

2 . Averbukh, E. S. Depressive states / E. S. Averbukh. - Л., 1962. - 134 с.

3 . Averbukh, E. S. Neuroses and neurosis-like states at a late age / E. S. Averbukh, M. E. Teleshevskaya. - Л., 1976. - 160 с.

4 . The Actual Problems of Suicidology. Moscow Research Institute of Psychiatry. V. Kovalev. - M., 1981. - T. 92. - 264 с.

5 . Antropov, Y. F. Clinical and pathogenetic features and therapy of somatized depression in children and adolescents / Y. F. Antropov // Ros. psikhiatr. zhurn. 1999. - № 1. - C. 7—11.

6 . Antropov, Y. F. Pathological habitual behaviors in children and adolescents / Y. F. Antropov, Y. S. Shevchenko. - M., 1999. - 304 с.

7 . F. Antropov. Neurotic Depression in Children and Adolescents (Clinic, Typology, Dynamics and Differential Therapy). - M. : Medpraktika, 2001. - 151 с.

8 . F. Antropov. Therapy of neurotic depression in children and adolescents / F. Antropov // Ros. psikhiatr. zhurn. 2001. - № 2. - C. 53—56.

9 . Anufriev, A. K. Hidden Endogenous Depressions. Message 2. Clinical symptomatology / A.K. Anufriev // Jour. of neuropathology and psychiatry. - 1970. - № 6. - C. 941—947.

10 . Bardenstein, L. M. Pathological heteroaggressive behavior in adolescents / L. M. Bardenstein, J. B. Mozhginsky. - M., 2000.

11 Batuev A. S., Sokolova L. V. The doctrine of dominant as a theoretical basis for the formation of the mother-child system / A. S. Batuev, L. V. Sokolova // Vestnik (Herald) of St. Petersburg State University. - 1994. - Vol. 2. - C. 82— 102.

12 Batuev, A. S. The emergence of the psyche in the prenatal period / A. S. Batuev // Psikholog. zhurn. 2000. - T. 21, № 6. - C. 51—56.

13 . Batygina, G. 3. Clinical features of depression and adolescence in the state of social orphanhood / G. 3. Batygina // Orphans of Russia: problems, hopes, future. - M., 1994. - C. 48—49.

14 Bauer, T. The mental development of the infant / T. Bauer. - M. : Publishing house "Progress", 1985. - 187 с.

15 . Bashina, V. M. Affective disorders (syndromes) in the clinic of schizophrenia in children / V. M. Bashina // Journal of Neuropathology and Psychiatry. - 1981. - Ò. 81, p. 10. - C. 1514—1518.

16 . Bashina, V. M. Features of early childhood schizophrenia proceeding with asthenoadynamic, adynamic and affective-catatonic attacks / V. M. Bashina, N. V. Simashkova // Journal of Neuropathology and Psychiatry. - 1989. - Ò. 83, p. 5. 69.

17 . Bashina, V. M. Affective disorders in children : a guide to psychiatry / V. M.

Bashina. - M. : Medicine, 1999. - T. 2. - C. 570—578.

18 . Berezantsev, A. Yu. Motivation of socially dangerous actions and its value in diagnostics of emotional-volitional and intellectual disorders and patients with oligophrenia and an estimation of their social danger / A. Yu. Berezantsev // Differential diagnostics of mental disorders. - M., 1991. - C. 11—14.

19 Bomba, I. Juvenile depression (epidemiological study) / I. Bomba // Journal of neuropathology and psychiatry. - 1987. - Vol. 10. - C. 1501— 1503.

20 Bokhan N. A., Butorina N. E., Krivulin E. N. Depressive reactions in penitentiary maladaptation in adolescents. - Chelyabinsk : Publishing house PIRS, 2006. - 206 c.

21 . Brekhman, G.I. Perinatal psychology / G.I. Brekhman // Bulletin of the Russian Association of Obstetricians and Gynecologists. Russian Association of Obstetricians and Gynecologists. - 1998. - № 4. - C. 49—52.

22 . Brutman, V. I. The dynamics of the psychological state of women during pregnancy and after childbirth / V. I. Brutman, G. G. Filippova, I. Yu. - 2002. - № 3. - C. 59—68.

23 . Burelov, E.A. The comparative study of affective, volitional and behavioral disorders in oligophrenia and early residual-organic states during the pubertal crisis / E.A.Burelov // Theoretical and organizational questions of forensic psychiatry. - M., 1980. - C. 140—148.

24 Butorina, N. E. Deprivation dysontogenesis and school desadaptation / N.E. Butorina, G.G. Butorin // Ros. psikhiatr. zhurn. 1999. - №3. - C. 17— 23.

25 . Butorina N. E., E. V. Malinina // Problems of deviant behavior of youth in modern society. - SPb. St. Petersburg NIPI named after V. M. Bekhterev, 2001. - C. 23.

26 Bykov, A.V. The role of pharmacoeconomics in improving the choice and use of drugs / A.V. Bykov, Yu.B. Belousov // IV Russian. B. Belousov // IV Russian National Congress. "Man and medicine": theses of reports - Moscow, 1997. - C. 312.

27 . Vandysh, V. V. To the problem of the nosological concept of organic and mental disorders / V. V. Vandysh, I. M. Parkhomenko // Ros. psychiatr. zhurn. - 1998. - № 2. - C. 11—15.

28 Vvedensky, I. N. Psychogenic reactions in oligophrenics / I. N. Vvedensky, M. S. Heif // Neuropathology and psychiatry. - M., 1940. - T. 9, vol. 7-8. - C. 38—53.

29 . Vertogradova, O. P. Depression (psychopathology, pathogenesis). - M., 1980.

30 . Vertogradova, O. P. Analysis of structure of depressive triad as a diagnostic and prognostic sign / O. P. Vertogradova, V. M. Voloshin // Jour. of neuropathology and psychiatry. - 1989. - Vol. 83, p. 1. - C. 1189— 1194.

31 . Vertogradova O. P. Anxiety-phobic disorders and depression / O. P. Vertogradova // Anxiety and obsessions / ed. by A. B. Smulevich. - M., 1998. - C. 113—131.

32 . Winnicott, D. V. Little Children and their Mothers / D. V. Winnicott. - M. : Independent firm Klass, 1998.

33 Vinokurova, A. I. On the manic-depressive psychosis and syndrome in children / A. I. Vinokurova // Neurology, psychiatry and psychohygiene. - 1955. - № 2. - C. 119, 193.

34 The diagnosis, typology and prognosis of adolescent depression: Author's dissertation.... D. in medical sciences / T. V. Vladimirova. - M., 1986.

35 Volgina, S. Y. The structure and features of mental disorders in adolescents born prematurely / S. Y. Volgina // Ros. psikhiatr. zhurn. 1997. - № 3. - C. 21—23.

36 Vostroknutov, N. V. Typology of delinquent behavior in children and adolescents: social and environmental, emotional and personal and Psychopathological risk factors / Vostroknutov N.V. // Social maladaptation: behavioral disorders in children and adolescents: proceedings of the Russian Scientific-Practical Conference - Moscow, 1996. - C. 21—29.

37 . Vrono, M. Sh. Schizophrenia in Children and Adolescents / M. Sh. Vrono. - M., 1971. - 128 c.

38 Gavrilova S.I. Psychopharmacological and antiepileptic drugs approved for use in Russia / ed. Gavrilova S.I., Gecht A.B., Hoffman A.G., Kokoin I.V.. - M., 2004. - 301 c.

39 Gaiduk, F. M. Delayed mental development of cerebral-organic genesis in children (multifactorial study) : Author's dissertation / F. M. Gaiduk. - Minsk, 1985. - 33 c.

40 .Gampion, A. Rational use of drugs and pharmacoeconomics / A. Gampion. - M., 1997. - C. 26.

41 Garbuzov, V. I. Nervous children / V. I. Garbuzov. - Л., 1980. - 174 c.

42 . Gerish, A. A. Endogenous somatized depression in primary school-age children : autoref. D. in medical sciences / A.A. Gerish. - M., 1995. - 20 c.

43 Gilyarovsky, V.A. Psychiatry / V.A. Gilyarovsky. - M., 1935.

44 Golik, A. N. Social psychiatry of orphanhood: clinical, organizational and preventive aspects / A. N. Golik // XII congress of psychiatrists of Russia (materials of the congress). - M., 1995. - C. 52—53.

45 Golik, A. H. Child abuse and comorbid mental disorders (social and psychiatric analysis) / A. N. Golik. N. Golik // Deti Rossii : Violence and Protection : Materials of All-Russian Scientific-Practical Conf. - M., 1997. - C. 37—39.

46 Gorinov, V. V. The role of decompensations in socially dangerous behavior of patients with oligophrenia / V. V. Gorinov // Prevention of socially dangerous actions of the mentally ill. - M., 1986. - C. 111—115.

47 V. V. Gorinov, V. V. Typology of psychogenic disorders in patients with oligophrenia (forensic-psychiatric aspect) / V. V. Gorinov, M. V. Usukina // Problems of the theory and organization of forensic-psychiatric examination. - M., 1989. - C. 102—109.

48 Grigoryeva, E. A. Comparative clinical and evaluation of Coaxil and Amitriptelin in the treatment of moderate and silent depression / E. A. Grigoryeva, A. A. Dyakov, G. A. Grifanov // V Ross. National Congress. "Man and medicine": theses of reports: Moscow, 1997. - С. 157.

49 Grineva I.M., A.A. Hoholeva, I.M. Some age peculiarities of neuroses / I.M. Grineva, A.A. Hoholeva // Vrachestvennoe delo. - 1989. - № 3. - С. 90—92.

50 . Gubsky Y. I. Drugs in psychopharmacology / Y. I. Gubsky, V. A. Shapovalova, I. I. Kutko, V. V. Shapovalova. - Kiev, 1997. - 282 c.

51 Gurieva, V. A. To study clinical features of psychopath-like schizophrenia in childhood and adolescence / V. A. Gurieva, V. J. Gindikija, M. P. Isachenkova // Journe neuropathology and psychiatry. - 1980. - Vol. 10. - С. 532—535.

52 Gurieva, V. A. Prolonged psychogenias in adolescents and their influence on the forming personality / V. A. Gurieva // Sots. i klin. psikhiatriya. - 1994. - Vol. 2. - С. 31—35.

53 Gurieva, V. A. Psychopathology of adolescence / V. A. Gurieva, V. J. Gindikin, V. J. Semke. - Tomsk, 1994. - 309 c.

54 Gurieva, V. A. The modern state of adolescent forensic psychiatry and ways to improve it / V. A. Gurieva // Prospects of development of adolescent social and forensic psychiatry. - Moscow, Khabarovsk, 1995. - Ч. 2. - С. 8—12.

55 Gurieva, V. A. Psychogenic disorders in children and adolescents / V. A. Gurieva. - M., 1996. - 207 c.

56 Gurieva, V.A. Problems of modern adolescent psychiatry, ed. by T.B. Dmitrieva, V.A. Gurieva. - M., 2001. - С. 8—15.

57 . Danilova L.Y. Peculiarities of the course of cyclothymic schizophrenia of pubertal age / L.Y. Danilova // Journal of Neurologopathology and Psychiatry. - 1986. - Vol. 10. - С. 1539—1543.

58 . Danilova L.Y. Psychopathological features of cyclothymic depressions in low-gradient schizophrenia in prepubertal and pubertal age / L.Y. Danilova // Journal of neuropathology and psychiatry. - 1985. - Ò. 85, p. 10. - С. 1521—1526.

59 . Child psychiatry : textbook / edited by E. G. Eidemiller - St. Petersburg. Peter, 2005. - 1120 c.

60 . Dzeruzhinskaya, N. A. Clinical dynamics and social characteristics of mentally retarded who have committed repeated socially dangerous acts (ODD) / N. A. Dzeruzhinskaya // Forensic and social psychiatry of the 1990s. - Kyiv, 1994. - Т. 1. - С. 164—165.

61 . Dmitrieva, T. B. To a question on differential diagnostics of depressive conditions at pubertal age / T. B. Dmitrieva // Jour. of neuropathology and psychiatry. - 1980. - Vol. 2. - С. 237—242.

62 . Dmitrieva, T. B. Psychogenic depression in adolescence and adolescence (clinic, pathogenesis and treatment) : autoref. Candidate of medical sciences / T. B. Dmitrieva. - M., 1981. - 17 c.

63 . Dmitrieva, T. B. Affective disorders in children and adolescents (literature

review) / T. B. Dmitrieva, E. V. Makushkin, M. A. Fedina // Psychopharmacotherapy. - 2001. - T. 3, № 5. - C. 15—24.

64 . Dozortseva E. G. Psychology of abnormal development in adolescence (criminological aspect) : autoref. Doctor in Psychology. - M., 2000. - 48 c.

65 . Evidence-Based Medicine. Annual International Handbook. Part 3: Children's diseases. - Moscow: MediaSphere, 2003. - Vol. 2. - 1194 c.

66 . Drapkin, B. 3. Psychotherapy of maternal love / B. 3. Drapkin. - M. : DeLiPrint, 2004.

67 . Durenheim, E. Suicide / E. Durenheim // Suicidology. Past and Present : The problem of suicide in the works of philosophers, sociologists, psychotherapists and artistic texts. - M. : The Cogito-Center, 2001. - C. 239—254.

68 . Zavadenko N. N. Neurological bases of attention deficit and hyperactivity disorder in children: doctoral thesis / N. N. Zavadenko. - M., 1999. - 34 c.

69 . Zakharov, A. I. Psychotherapy of neuroses in children and teenagers. - Л., 1982. - 216 c.

70 . Iovchuk N. M. Depressive and manic states in children and adolescents / N. M. Iovchuk // Journal of Neuropathology and Psychiatry. - 1976. - Issue. 6. - C. 922—934.

71 . Iovchuk, N. M. Clinical and dynamic study of pubertal psychoses with affective cyclothymic debut / N. M. Iovchuk, V. G. Koziulia // Journal of Neuropathology and Psychiatry. - 1981. - Vol. 10. - C. 1509—1514.

72 . Iovchuk N. M. Clinical features of children's endogenous depression / N. M. Iovchuk // Problems of schizophrenia of childhood and adolescence. - M., 1986. - C. 61.

73 . Iovchuk, N. M. Endogenous affective disorders in childhood : autoref. D. in medical sciences / N.M. Iovchuk. - M., 1989. - 47 c.

74 . Iovchuk N. M. Depression in children and adolescents / N. M. Iovchuk, A. A. Severny. - M. : Shkola-Press, 1999. - 405 c.

75 . Iovchuk, N. M. Depression in the school adolescent population / N. M. Iovchuk, G. 3. Batygina // Ros. psikhiatr. zhurn. 1999. - № 3. - C. 37—40.

76 . Iovchuk N. M. To the problem of didactogenic disorders in schoolchildren / N. M. Iovchuk, A. A. Severny // Problems of mental health of children and teenagers (Scientific and practical journal of psychiatry, psychology, psychotherapy and related disciplines). - 2007. - № 2. - C. 9—17.

77 Isaev, D. N. Mental underdevelopment in children / D. N. Isaev. - Л., 1982. - 224 c.

78 Isayev, D. N. Psychoprophylaxis in the practice of the pediatrician / D. N. Isayev. - Л. Medicine, 1984. - 192 c.

79 Psychology of a sick child / D. N. Isaev. - SPb. : PPMI, 1993. - 76 c.

80 Isaev, D. N. Psychosomatic medicine of childhood / D. N. Isaev. - SPb., 1993.

81 Kalashnikova, A. A. The system "mother-child" as a corrective factor in hospital conditions for children of preschool age // the Congress of psychiatrists of Russia (materials of the congress) / A. A. Kalashnikova, I. N.

Tatarova, J. B. Kovalenko. - M., 1995. - C. 384—385.

82 M. A. Kalinina, N. I. Golubeva // Problems of deviant behavior of youth in modern society. - Saint-Petersburg. V. M. Bekhterev Research Institute, St. Petersburg, 2001. - C. 52.

83 Kalinina, M. A. On the mental consequences of raising children and teenagers in conditions of orphanhood / M. A. Kalinina, M. E. Proselkova // Social maladaptation: behavioural disorders in children and teenagers. - M., 1996. - C. 110.

84 . Kashnikova, A.A. Psychopathic equivalents of depression in children and adolescents / A.A. Kashnikova, O.D. Sosyukalo, I.N. Tatarova // Journal of Neuropathology and Psychiatry. - 1983. - 1983. 10. - C. 1522—1526.

85 Kim, L. V. Depressive disorders among teenagers : socio-psychological features / L. V. Kim // Questions of mental health of children and teenagers (Scientific and practical journal of psychiatry, psychology, psychotherapy and related disciplines. - 2006 (6). - № 2. - C. 122—129.

86 Clinical and forensic adolescent psychiatry / V. A. Gurieva, T. B. Dmitrieva, E. V. Makushkin et al. Ed. by V.A. Gurieva. A. Gurieva. - Moscow. : Medical Information Agency, 2007. - 488 c.

87 Kovalev, V. V. Psychiatry of childhood / V. V. Kovalev. - M., 1979. - 607 c.

88 Kovalev, V. V. Semiotics and diagnostics of mental diseases in children and adolescents / V. V. Kovalev. - M. : Medicine, 1985. - 286 c.

89 Kovalev, V. V. Psychiatry of childhood: handbook for doctors / V. V. Kovalev. - M. : Medicine, 1995. - 560 c.

90 . Kozidubova V. M. Depression in adolescents (clinic, psychopatholgypnye features, questions of pathogenesis) : autoref. D. in Medicine / V.M. Kozidubova. - M., 1992. - 51 c.

91 Kozlova I.A. Schizophrenia in childhood and adolescence : a handbook on psychiatry / I.A. Kozlova. - M. : Medicine, 1999. -T. 2. - C. 472—487.

92 Kozlovskaya, G. V. Emotional disorders in the conditions of orphanhood in young children. Orphans of Russia: Problems, Hopes, Future / G. V. Kozlovskaya, M. E. Proselkova. - M., 1994. - C. 55—57.

93 Kozlovskaya, G. V. Micropsychiatry and possibilities of correction of mental disorders in infancy / G. V. Kozlovskaya, O. V. Bazhenova // Jour. of neurology and psychiatry. - 1995. - Vol. 5. - C. 48—51.

94 . Kolotilin, G.F. Depressive states at teenagers / G.F. Kolotilin // Materials of the 3rd All-Russia conf. on neurology and psychiatry of childhood. - M., 1971. - C. 155—157.

95 Konovalova, V. V. Depressive disorders in mentally retarded children / V. V. Konovalova, T. A. Kupriyanova, T. N. Prilepskaya // Mental disorders in childhood and adolescence. - 2003. - C. 121—122.

96 Kornilov, A. A. Attraction disorders in children and adolescents / A. A. Kornilov, E. S. Vishnevskaya, N. P. Kokorina // Siberian Bulletin of Psychiatry and Narcology. - 2003. - № 3 (29). - C. 52—53.

97 . Kryzhanovskaya I. L. On variants of the cerebrasthenic syndrome in mentally retarded children / I. L. Kryzhanovskaya // Ros. psikhiatr. zhurn. 1999. - № 3. - C. 40—43.

98 The psychopath-like states in the main psychiatric diseases of adolescence : autoref. diss. D. in medical sciences / A. S. Kurashov. - M., 2001. - 48 c.

99 . Langmeier, J. Mental Deprivation in   childhood / J. Langmeyer, 3. Matejček. - Prague : Avitsenum, 1984. - 334 c.

100. Lapides, M. I. Questions of child psychiatry / M. I. Lapides. - M., 1940. - C. 39—76.

101. Lebedinsky, V. V. Violations of mental development in children: Textbook / V. V. Lebedinsky. - M. : MGSHU, 1985. - 167 c.

102. Lebedinsky, V. V. Emotional disorders in childhood and their correction / V. V. Lebedinsky. - M., 1990. - 197 c.

103. Lichko A. E. Psychopathy and accentuations of character in adolescents / A. E. Licko. - Л., 1983. - 255 c.

104. Lichko, A. E. Adolescent psychiatry / A. E. Lichko. - Л., 1985. -416 c.

105. Lomachenkov, A. S. On the diagnosis and prognosis of MDP in children and adolescents // Proceedings of the Leningrad Medical Institute / A. S. Lomachenkov. - Л., 1971. - T. 57.

106. Lopatina, O. G. The value of physical contact with the mother in the prevention of behavioral disorders in the child / O. G. Lopatina // Social and clinical psychiatry. - 1992. - T. 2, № 2. - C. 79—82.

107. Loskutova,   E.   E.   Methodological problems of conducting Pharmacological study / E.E. Loskutova // V Ros. National Congress. "Man and medicine" : theses of reports - Moscow - 1998. - C. 699.

108. Loskutova E. E., Maksimkina E.A., Dorouchiva V.V. Modeling the Efficiency of Allocations for Drug Assistance to the Mentally Ill / E. E. Loskutova, E.A. Maksimkina, V.V. Dorouchiva // II Ros. National Congress. "The man and the medicine" : theses of reports - Moscow, 1995. - C. 9.

109. Loskutova, E. E. Theoretical bases of pharmaceutical economy / E. E. Loskutova // Formation of drug policy priorities : theses of reports - Moscow, 1995. - C. 29.

110. Loskutova,   E. E. The direction of applied research on Pharmaceutical economy / E.E. Loskutova // V Ros. National Congress. "Man and medicine" : theses of reports - Moscow, 1997. - C. 320.

111. The Psychopharmacology of Children and Adolescents / I. A. Lvov. - SPb., 1993. - C. 9.

112. Makushkin, E. V. Clinical and evolutionary systematics and forensic and psychiatric significance of dysontogenetic mental disorders in adolescents : autoref. D. in medical sciences / E.V. Makushkin. - M., 2002. - 52 c.

113. Mamtseva, V. N. Depressive neurosis in childhood / V. N. Mamtseva. - M., 1982.

114. Mamtseva, V.N. One of variants of the masked depression with hyperthermia at schizophrenia at children / V.N.Mamtseva // Jour. of neuropathology and psychiatry. - 1988. - Vol. 10. - C. 57—62.

115. Modina, A. I. Development of emotions in young children / A. I. Modina. - M., 1971. - 32 c.

116. B. Mozhginsky // Borderline disorders in forensic psychiatric practice: collection of scientific works / ed. by T. B. Dmitrieva. - M., 1991. - C. 3—7.

117. B. Mozhginsky // Differential diagnostics of mental disorders. - M., 1991. - C. 50.

118. Mozhginsky, Y. B. Affective disorders in the structure of adolescent psychopathic-like syndromes : autoref. d. ... B. Mozhginsky. - M., 1993. - 18 c.

119. In the case of the psychogenic personality development of minors, the acute affective reactions of the minors: dissertation.... Cand. medical sciences / N.B. Morozova. - M., 1986. - 21 c.

120. *In the* case of the psychopathological assessment of the psychogenic development of personality in the juvenile population, the following is presented as a method of instruction. - M., 1990. - 15 c.

121. Morozova, N.B. Children and sexual abuse / N.B. Morozova // Differential diagnostics of mental disorders. - M., 1991. - C. 83—85.

122. Mosolov, S. N. Clinical application of antidepressants / S. N. Mosolov. - SPb., 1995. - 366 c.

123. Mosolov, S. N. Fundamentals of psychopharmacotherapy. - M., 1996. - 100 c.

124. Mukhamedrakhimov, R. J. Forms of interaction between a mother and an infant / R. J. Mukhamedrakhimov // Voprosy psychologii. - 1994. - № 6. - C. 16—25.

125. Mukhamedrakhimov, R. J. Interaction and attachment of mothers and infants of risk groups / R. J. Mukhamedrakhimov // Voprosy psychologii. - 1998. - № 2. - C. 18—33.

126. Mukhamedrakhimov, R. J. Mother and Infant; Psychological interaction / R. J. Mukhamedrakhimov. - SPb. : Speech, 2003.

127. Mukhin, S. S. The clinical picture of manic-depressive psychosis in children / S. S. Mukhin // Soviet neuropsychiatry. - Л., 1940. - VOL. III. - C. 34—48.

128. Natalevich, E.S. Psychogenic depressions in adolescence / E.S. Natalevich, V.D. Koroleva, L.I. Kuryndina, V.I. Posokhova // Psychogenic diseases and problems of deontology in forensic psychiatric practice. - M., 1982. - C. 57—67.

129. Nikolaev Y. M. Psychoneurological predictors of deviant behavior in adolescent girls with residual-organic brain damage / M. Nikolaev // Ros. psikhiatr. zhurn. 1998. - № 4. - C. 42—44.

130. Nuller, Y.L. Affective psychoses / Y.L. Nuller. - Л., 1988.

131. Ozeretskiy, N. I. Psychopathology of childhood / N. I. Ozeretskiy. - M. : Uchpedgiz, 1938.

132. Ozertskovsky, S. D. On latent endogenous depressions in adolescents / S. D. Ozertskovsky // Journal of Neuropathology and Psychiatry. - 1979. - Vol. 2. - C. 212.

133. Ozeretskovsky, S. D. Depressive states in the clinic of schizophrenia in adolescents / S.D. Ozeretskovsky // 8th All-Union Congress of neuropathologists, psychiatrists and narcologists. - M., 1988. - T. 2. - C. 364.

134. Oleichik, I. V. Depressive disorders with the syndrome of youth asthenic insolvency : autoref. diss. Candidate of medical sciences / I. V. Oleichik. - M., 1998.

135. Panteleeva, G. P. Affective psychosis / G. P. Panteleeva // Manual on psychiatry. - 1999. - T. 1. - C. 555—578.

136. Papadopoulos, T. F. Handbook of Psychiatry / T. F. Papadopoulos. - M., 1983. - T. 1. - C. 417—456.

137. Parashchenko, A. F. Therapy of schizophrenia by seroquel in child psychiatric practice / A. F. Parashchenko, B. Barynikov, M. B. Kotina, Kashichkina et al. B. Barynikov, M.B. Kotina, Kashichkina et al. // Topical questions of child psychiatry: Materials of the All-Russian Scientific-Practical Conference: Saratov, 2006. - C. 7.

138. Parkhomenko E.V. Cost-effectiveness analysis in analgesic therapy with tramal / E.V. Parkhomenko, E.E. Loskutova // V Ross. National Congress. "Man and medicine": theses of reports: Moscow, 1998. - C. 706.

139. Petrov, L.A. Reactive conditions arising in retarded children, their influence on the resolution of sanity issues and peculiarities of the course of these reactive states / L.A. Petrov // Problems of forensic psychiatry. - M., 1960. - C. 164—169.

140. Pivovarova G.N. About reactive depressions at children and teenagers. - M., 1956.

141. Pletnev, D. D. To a question about somatic cyclothymia / D. D. Pletnev // Russian Clinic. - 1927. - T. 7, № 36. - C. 496.

142. Adolescent forensic psychiatry / ed. by V. A. Gurieva. A. Gurieva // Guidance for doctors. - M., 1996.

143. V. Popov // Self-destructive behavior in adolescents: Collection of articles / ed. by A. E. Lichko, V. V. Popov. - Л., 1991. - C. 5—9.

144. Posokhova V. I. Clinical forms of psychogenic depressions in adolescence and adolescence and their forensic psychiatric assessment : autoref. Candidate of medical sciences / V.I. Posokhova. - M., 1982. - 20 c.

145. Practice of forensic psychiatric examination / E.V. Makushkin, S.V. Kuderinov, M.V. Morozova, E.S. Ambartsumyan. - M., 2001. - Sb. 39. - C. 5—20.

146. Prashchenko A. F. Peculiarities of olanzapine administration in juveniles suffering from schizophrenia / A. F. Prashchenko, Yu.

Barylnik // Topical issues of child psychiatry: materials of the All-Russian Scientific-Practical Conference - Saratov, 2006. - C. 73.

147. Psychiatry of childhood and adolescence / edited by K. Gillberg, L. Hellgren / edited by P. I. Sidorov; translated from Sweden. A. Makkoveeva. - MOSCOW: GEOTAR-MED, 2004. - 544 c.

148. Psychiatry and economic policy in health care / V.S. Yastrebov, V.P. Korchagin, T.A. Solokhina et al. Social and Clinical Psychiatry. - 1995. - T. 5, № 2. - C. 109—114.

149. Puzyreva, E. A. Family factors in the formation of inorganic enuresis in children 5-12 years old / E. A. Puzyreva // Problems of deviant behavior in modern society. - Saint-Petersburg. Saint-Petersburg scientifically-research institution named after V.M. Bekhterev, 2001. - C. 83.

150. Regional cerebral and systemic hemodynamic disorders in hypoxic-traumatic brain injury in preterm infants / I. Kravtsov, A.I. Egorova, G.P. Serebrennikova, R.D. Shadrina, L.I. Perepletchikova // Pediatrics. - 1988. - № 7. - C. 13— 16.

151. Savostyanova O. L. Anxiety-phobic disorders in childhood : autoref. diss. D. in medical sciences / O.L. Savostyanova. - M., 2001. - 378 c.

152. Salovsky, M.M. Rational use of medicines on the basis of territorial formulary system / M.M. Salovsky // V Ros. National Congress. "Man and medicine" : theses. of reports - Moscow, 1997. - C. 338.

153. Samarina, E. I. Clinical analysis of the structure of pupils of a boarding school for children with severe mental retardation / E. I. Samarina // Voprosy Mental Health of Children and Teenagers (Scientific and Practical Journal of Psychiatry, Psychology, Psychotherapy and Allied Disciplines. - 2007 (7). - № 1. - C. 18—27.

154. Sakharov, E.A. Age-specific psychological crises as pre-dosological forms of mental disorders in children and teenagers / E.A. Sakharov // Ros. psikhiatr. zhurn. 1997. - № 2. - C. 44—46.

155. Sboeva S.G. Development of pharmaceutical economy concept / S.G. Sboeva, E.E. Loskutova // IV Ros. National Congress. "Man and medicine": theses. of reports - Moscow, 1997. - C. 338.

156. Northern,   A. A.   The Principles of Disguising Masked A. Severny // Topical issues of neurology, psychiatry and neurosurgery: Proceedings of the 2nd Congress of neurologists, psychiatrists and neurosurgeons of the Latvian Soviet Socialist Republic. - Riga, 1985. - T. 1. - C. 169.

157. Severny, A.A. Endogenous depression / A.A. Severny. - Irkutsk, 1992. - C. 84—85.

158. Sergeev I. I. Peculiarities of hypochondriacal conditions in children and adolescents / I. I. Sergeev, V. I. Borodin // Journal of Neuropathology and Psychiatry. - 1991. - Vol. 8. - C. 32—34.

159. Serdyukovskaya, G. N. Psychohygiene of children and adolescents / G. N.

Serdyukovskaya. - M., 1985. - C. 7—16.

160. Simson, T. P. Neuroses in children, their prevention and treatment / T. P. Simson. - M., 1958. - C. 89—95.

161. Smirnova E. O. Development of the attachment theory / E. O. Smirnova, R. P. Radeeva // Voprosy psychologii. - 1998. - № 1. - C. 105—116.

162. Depression in general medical practice / A.B.Smulevich. - M.: Publishing house "Bereg", 2000. - 160 c.

163. Depression and comorbid disorders / A.B.Smulevich. - M., 1997.

164. Smulevich, A. B. To the epidemiological characteristic of patients with anxious-phobic disorders / A. B. Smulevich et al. (in Russian) // Anxiety and obsessions. - M., 1998. - C. 54—65.

165. Smulevich, N.A. Reactive depression of late age, its typology, course and results in a comparative-age aspect / N.A.Smulevich // Jour. of neuropathology and psychiatry. - 1989. - Vol. 4. - C. 76—82.

166. Snezhnevsky, A. V. Guide to Psychiatry / A. V. Snezhnevsky. - M., 1968.

167. Solokhina T.A. Financing of psychiatric hospitals on the basis of clinical and statistical groups / T.A. Solokhina, L.S. Shevchenko, E.G. Rytnik et al. // Sotsial'naya i klinicheskaya psikhiatriya. - 1993. - T 3, № 3. - C. 47—53.

168. Sosyukalo O. D. Psychopathic equivalents of depression in children and adolescents / O. D. Sosyukalo, A. A. Kashnikova, I. N. Tatarova // Journal of Neuropathology and Psychiatry. - 1983. - 1983. 10. - C. 1522.

169. Sosyukalo O. D. Affective pathology in children and the problem of deviant behavior / O. D. Sosyukalo // Topical issues of neurology and psychiatry of childhood: Tashkent, 1984. - C. 187—189.

170. Sukhareva, G. E. Some statements on principles of schizophrenic diagnostics / G. E. Sukhareva // Problems of children's psychiatry. - M., 1949. - C. 5—27.

171. Sukhareva, G. E. Clinical lectures on psychiatry of childhood / G. E. Sukhareva. - M., 1955. - T. 1—2. - 458 c.

172. Sukhareva, G. E. Clinical lectures on psychiatry of childhood / G. E. Sukhareva. - M., 1965. - C. 360—456.

173. Sukhareva, G.E. The role of age factor in the clinic of childhood psychoses / G.E. Sukhareva // Jour. of neuropathology and psychiatry. - 1970. - Vol. 10. - C. 1513—1516.

174. Sukhareva G. E. Lectures on Psychiatry of Childhood (selected chapters) / G. E. Sukhareva. - M. : Medicine, 1974. - 320 c.

175. Tabachnikov, A. E. Conditions of formation of boundary mental disorders in students of schools of a new type / A. E. Tabachnikov // Ros. psikhiatr. zhurn. - 1998. - № 1. - C. 36—39.

176. Tatarova I. N. Psychopathic equivalents of depression in schizophrenia in children and adolescents : autoref. diss. D. in medical sciences / Tatarova I.N.. - M., 1985. - C. 20.

177. The prevalence of mental disorders among children, adolescents and young people in the Russian Federation in 1991-1995 / N.A. Tworogova // Ros. psikhiatr. zhurn. - 1997. - № 2. - C. 46—52.

178. Tiganov, A. S. Masked depression / A. S. Tiganov, L. N. Vidmanova, T. P. Platonova, A. A. Sukhonsky // Clinical Medicine. - 1986. - T. 64, № 9. - C. 6—11.

179. Tiganov A. S. Endogenous Depressions: Issues of Classification and Systematics. Depression and comorbid disorders / A.S. Tiganov. - M., 1997. - C. 12—26.

180. Tiganov, A. S. Guide to Psychiatry / A. S. Tiganov. - M. 1999. - C. 542.

181. Ustyugova A.M., Solonina A.V., Rostova N.B. Analysis of the effectiveness of the use of funds for the procurement of drugs for the therapy of newborns / A.M. Ustyugova, A.V., Rostova N.B. // V Ros. Nat. congr. "Man and medicine": theses. of reports: Moscow, 1998. - C. 714.

182. Ushakov, G.K. Children's psychiatry / G.K. Ushakov. - M., 1973. -321 c.

183. Pharmacoeconomic aspects of treatment of depressive states with paxilon / I. L. Gurovich, A. B. Shenooksher, A. I. Aldonin et al. / / Social and clinical psychiatry. - 1998. - № 3. - C. 55—62.

184. Felinskaya, N. I. Oligophrenia / N. I. Felinskaya // Forensic psychiatry. - M., 1950. - C. 258—271.

185. Fel, M. I. Neurotic Depressions in Adolescents / M. I. Fel // Voprosy psychoneurology. - Baku, 1982. - T. 9. - C. 311—313.

186. Filippova, G. G. Maternity: a comparative approach / G. G. Filippova // Psycholog. zhurn. - 1999. - T. 20, № 5. - C. 81—88.

187. Filippova, G. G. Psychology of motherhood / G. G. Filippova. - Moscow: Institute of Psychotherapy, 2002.

188. Frayerov, O. E. Mild degrees of oligophrenia (retardation). Clinic and Examination / O. E. Freierov. - Moscow : Medicine, 1964. - 224 c.

189. Frolov B. S. New control over the course of depression to prevent suicidal behavior / B. S. Frolov, I. V. Ovechkina // Problems of deviant youth behavior in modern society. - SPb. Saint-Petersburg NIPI named after V. M. Bekhterev, 2001. - C. 102—103.

190. Kharitonova N.K., Posokhova V.I. Psychogenically provoked depressive syndromes in the initial stages of schizophrenia in adolescents / N.K. Kharitonova. - M., 1983. - C. 71—73.

191. Kharitonova N. K. Psychogenic depressions (systematics, principles of modeling, forensic-psychiatric value) : autoref. Doctor of Medicine / N.K. Kharitonova. - M., 1991. - 46 c.

192. Khoroshko, V.K. Suicide in children / V.K. Khoroshko // Ros. psikhiatr. zhurn. - 1998. - № 3. - C. 70—80.

193. Tsaregradskaya, J.V. The child from conception to one year / J.V. Tsaregradskaya. - M. : AST, 2002.

194. The clinical picture and differential diagnostic estimation of some

psychopathological syndromes of puberty age / M.J.Tsutsulkovsky, G.P.Panteleyeva // Problems of schizophrenia of children and teenagers. - M., 1986. - C. 13—15.

195. Tsutsulkovskaya, M. J. The premorbid personality of patients with adolescent attack-like schizophrenia / M. J. Tsutsulkovskaya, V. A. Mikhailova // Journal of Neuropathology and Psychiatry. - 1977. - Vol. 4. - C. 547—557.

196. Chekhova, A. N. The course of the schizophrenic process, which began in childhood / A. N. Chekhova. - M., 1968. - 136 c.

197. V. F. Shalimov, Novikova G. R. Results of complex medical and psychological examination of children of the senior preschool age who are in conditions of family deprivation / V. F. Shalimov, G. R. Novikova // Problems of deviant behavior of youth in modern society. - SPb. Saint-Petersburg NIPI named after V. M. Bekhterev, 2001. - C. 111.

198. Shevchenko, Y. S. Problems of mental health care for children and adolescents / Y. S. Shevchenko, N. M. Iovchuk. - M., 1998. - C. 37—39.

199. Shchukina, E. G. Features of Families Raising Children with disabilities : ways of solving / E. G. Shchukina // Modern Family : problems, ways of formation and development : collection of articles. - Arkhangelsk : SGMU, 2003. - C. 18—20.

200. Shchukina E. G. The role of the family in the process of waiting for a child / E. G. Shchukina // Problems of prenatal psychology : a method manual. - Arkhangelsk : SGMU, 2003. - C. 5—10.

201. Yusevich L. S. Forensic psychiatric assessment of organic lesions of the central nervous system in minors / L. S. Yusevich // Problems of forensic psychiatry. - M., 1946. - Sb. 5. - C. 325—355.

202. Adewuya, A. O. Factors associated with depressive symptoms in Nigerian adolescents / A. O. Adewuya // J. Child Abuse Negl. - 2006. - Jun. - P. 15.

203. Ajuriaguerra, J. D Psychiatric de l'enfant / J. D. Ajuriaguerra. - Paris : Masson, 1970. - 1023 p.

204. Ajuriaguerra, J. Manuel de psychiartie de l'enfant / J. Ajuriaguerra. - Paris, 1970. - P. 701—714.

205. Albert, N. Incidence of depression in early adolescence / N. Albert, A. T. Beck // J. Youth. Adol. - 1975. - V. 4, № 4. - P. 301-307.

206. Alderman, J. / J. Alderman, R. Wolkov, M. Chung et al. Acad. Child Adolesc. Psychiatry. - 1998. - Vol. 37. - P. 386—394.

207. Altschulova, J. Psychiatric Aspects of the Asthma-Eczema Syndrome in Children and Young People with Special Reference to Depression / J. Altschulova // Depressive States in Childhood and Adolescence. - Stockholm, 1972. - P. 193—196.

208. Amon, P. Intelligence and language performance of special education children at 7 and 9 years of age / P. Amon et al. // Prax. Kinderpsychol.

Kinderpsychiatr. - 1995. - Jul. - № 4416. - P. 196—203.

209. Annell, A. L. Depressive States in Childhood and Adolescence / Annell A. L. // Depressive States in Childhood and Adolescence. - Stockholm, 1972. - P. 11— 15.

210. Anthony, Y. Manic-depressive psychosis in childhood / Y. Anthony, P. Scott // J. Child. Psychol. Psychiatr. - 1960. - V. 1, № 1. - P. 53-61.

211. Asperger, H. Handbuch der Kinderheilkunde / hrsg. H. Opitz, F. Schmid / H. Asperger. - Berlin, 1969.

212. Avci, A. Comparison of moclobemide and placebo in young adolescents with major depressive disorder / A. Avci, R. S. Diler, M. Kibar, F. Sezgin // Ann. Med. Sci. - 1999. - V. 8. - P. 31—40.

213. Baeyer von W. Depreesionszuatande in kindheit und Juged / W. von Baeyer // The depressive syndrome / edited by H. Hippins, H. Selbsch. - Munchen, Berlin, Wien : Urban et Schwarzenberg, 1969. - pp. 361-378.

214. Ballenger, J. C. Biological aspects of depression : Implications for clinical practice / J. C. Ballenger // Review of psychiatry /eds. A. J. Fraces, R. E. Hales. - Washington : Am. Psychiatric Press, 1988. - P. 169—187.

215. Bandura, A. Social learning theory / A. Bandura. - Englewood Cliffs : Prentice-Hall, 1977.

216. Barbe, R. P. Clinical differences between suicidal and nonsuicidal depressed children and adolescents / R. P. Barbe, D. E. Williamson, J. A. Bridge // J. Clin. Psychiatry. - 2005. - Apr. - V. 66, № 4. - P. 492-498.

217. Bauersfeld, K. H. Diagnosis and treatment of depressive states in a school psychiatric outreach clinic / K. H. Bauersfeld // Depressive States in Childhood and Adolescence. - Stockholm, 1972. p. 281-285.

218. Beck, A. T. Cognitive therapy and the emotional disorders / A. T. Beck. - N. Y. : Internat. Univ. Press, 1976.

219. Beier, D. C. Behavioral disturbances in the mentally retarded / D. C Beier // Mental retardation / eds. H. A. Stevens, R. Huber. - Chicago, 1964. - 615 p.

220. Bender, L. Psychopathology of schizophrenia / L. Bender. - New York, London, 1966. - 354 p.

221. Biederman, J. A controlled longitudinal 5-year follow-up study of children at high and low risk for panic disorder and major depression / J. Biederman // J. Nerv. Ment. Dis. - 2006. - May. - V. 194, № 5. - P. 382-385.

222. Biermann, I. A case of infantile cyclothymia with special familial stress / I. Biermann, B. Pflug // Acta paedopsychiat. - 1974. V. 40, № 5. P. 196-202.

223. Blanchard, L. T. Emotional, developmental, and behavioral health of American children and their families : a report from the 2003 National Survey of Children's Health / Blanchard L. T. // Alcohol. Clin. Exp. Res. - 2006. - Jun. - V. 30, № 6. - P. 1051-1059.

224. Bomba, J. Rozpwzechnievie i obraz depression u dzieci i modzieri w ssietle bezposiernich badania populacji niele leczenia / J. Bomba, W. Badura-Madej,

Bielska et al. // Psychiat. Pol. - 1986. - V. 20, № 3. - P. 184.

225. Bortnick-Duffy, S. A. Who are the dually diagnosed? / S. A. Bortnick-Duffy, R. K. Eyman // Am. J. Ment. Retard. - 1990. - V. 94, № 6. - P. 586.

226. Bradley, C. Definition of childhood in psychiatric literature / C. Bradley // Am. J. Psychiatry. - 1937. - V. 94, № 1. - P. 33-36.

227. Breier, A. The diagnostic validity of anxiety disorders and their relationship to depressive illness / A. Breier, D. S. Charney, G. R. Heninger // Am. J. Psychiatry. - 1985. - V. 142. - P. 787—797.

228. Brent, D. A. Psychiatric risk factors for adolescent suicide : A case-control study / D. A. Brent, J. A. Perper, G. Moritz, C. Allman et. Al. // J. of the Amercan Academi of Child and Adolescent Psychiatry. - 1993. - V. 32. - P. 521—529.

229. Brent, D. Psychoeducational program for families of affectively ill children and adolescents / D. Brent, K. Poling, B. McKain, M. Baugher // J. Am. Acad. Child. Adolesc. Psychiatry. - 1993. - V. 32. - P. 770—774.

230. Brown, W. A. Response to dexamethasone and subtype of depression / W. A. Brown, I. Shuey // Arch. Gen. Psychiat. - 1980. - V. 37. - P. 747—751.

231. Bruch, H. Uber die psychologischen Aspekte der Fettleibigkeit / H. Bruch // Med. clin. - 1960. - V. 55. - p. 295.

232. Brummelte, S. High post-partum levels of corticosterone given to dams influence postnatal hippocampal cell proliferation and behavior of spring : A model of post-partum stress and possible depression / S. Brummelte // J. Infect. Dis. - 2006. - Jul. - V. 194, № 2. - P 247-25.

233. Butefish, C. Neurological features of perinatal study of a neonate with multicystic encephalopathy / C. Butefish et al. // Semin. Pediatr. Neurol. - 1996. - Sep. - V. 3, № 3. - P. 236-242.

234. Butler, L. The effect of two school-based intervention programs on depressive symptoms in preadolescents / L. Butler et al. // Am. Educat. Researh J. - 1980. - V. 17. - P. 111—119.

235. Campbell, J. D. Manic-depressive psychosis in children. Report of 18 cases / J. D. Campbell // J. Nerv. Ment. Dis. - 1952. - V. 116, № 11. - P. 424.

236. Cantwell, D. P. Childhood Depression : What Do We Know, where Do We Go? / D. P. Cantwell // Childhood psychopathology and development / ed. S. B. Guse, F. J. Earls, J. E. Barrett. - New York : Raven Press, 1983. - 307 p.

237. Carlson, G. A. Unmasking masked depression in children and adolescent / G. A. Carlson, D. P. Cantwell // Am. J. Psychiat. - 1980. - V. 137. - P. 445—449.

238. Carlson, G. A. Suicidal behavior and depression in children and adolescents / G. A. Carlson, D. P. Cantwell // J. Am. Acad. Child. Psychiatr. - 1982. - V. 21, № 4. - P. 361-368.

239. Carlson, G. A. Development issues in the classification of depression in children / G. A. Carlson, J. Garber // Depression in young people / eds. M.

Rutter, C. Izard, P. Read. - N. Y. : Guilford, 1986.

240. Caron, C. Comorbidity in child psychopathology : Concepts issuis and research strategies / C. Caron, M. Rutter // J. Child Psychol. And Psychiatr. - 1991. - V. 32. - P. 1063—1080.

241. Cassullo, A. G. The role of depression in the dynamic process of obsessive disorders in childhood / A. G. Cassullo, M. E. Fabiani // Depressive States in Childhood and Adolescence. - Stockholm, 1972. - P. 233—238.

242. Cheung, A. H. The use of antidepressants to treat depression in children and adolescents / A. H. Cheung, G. J. Emslie, T. L. Mayes // Can. Med. Association J. - 2006. - Jan. - V. 174, № 2. - P. 193-200.

243. Chwast, J. Depressive reactions as manifested among adolescent delinquents / J. Chwast // Am. J. Psychotherapy. - 1967. - V. XXI. - P. 575—584.

244. Cicchetti, D. An organizational approach to childhood depression / D. Cicchetti, K. Schneider-Rosen // Depression in young people / eds. M. Rutter, C. Izard, P. Read. - N. Y. : Guilford, 1986.

245. Connell, H. M. Depression in Childhood / H. M. Connell // J. Child Psychiat., Hurn. Developm. - 1972. - V. 4. - P. 71—85. .

246. Corboz, R. Depressionen bei psychoorganisch gestorten Kindern / R. Gorboz // Depressive States in Childhood and Adolescence. - Stockholm, 1972. - P. 239— 249.

247. Costello, E. J. Psychiatric disorders in pediatric primary care / E. J. Costello, A. J. Costello, B. J. Burns, M. K. Dulcan, D. Brent, S. Janiszewski // Arch. Gen. Psychiatry. - 1988. - V. 45. - P. 1107—1116.

248. Craighead, W. E. A brief clinical history of cognitive-behavior therapy with children / W. E. Craighead // School. Psychol. Rev. - 1982. - V. 11. - P. 5—13.

249. Craighead, W. E. Away from a unitary model of depression / W. E. Craighead // Behav. Therapy. - 1980. - V. 11. - P. 122—128.

250. Cwast, J. Depressive reactions as manifested among adolescent delinquents / J. Cwast // Am. J. Psychotherapy. - 1967. - V. XXI. - P. 575—584.

251. Cytryn, L. Proposed classification of childhood depression / L. Cytryn, D. H. McKnew // Am. J. Psychiat. - 1972. - V. 129, № 2. - P. 149-155.

252. Delasiauve La note en J. l'Experience, 1840, Delasiauve La note en Gazette des hopitaux, 1852, Delasiauve Notes sur les fievres intermittentes, 1854, Delasiauve Revue en // J. De med. Mentale. - 1864. - P. 262.

253. De Veaugh-Geiss, J. Child and adolescent psychopharmacology in the new millennium : a workshop for academia, industry, and government / J. DeVeaugh- Geiss, J. March, M. Shapiro et al. // J. Am. Acad. Child. Adolesc. Psychiatry. - 2006. - Mar. - V. 45, № 3. - P. 261-270.

254. Dittmann, R. W. Olanzapine in adolescent and young adult patients with schizophrenia : Does subjective well-being improve? European

Neuropsychopharmacology / R. W. Dittmann, U. Hagenah, J. Junghan // The J. of the European College of Neuropsychopharmacology. - 2004. - V. 14. - Suppl. 3. - P. 296.

255. Donnelly, C. L. Efficacy and safety of sertraline in the treatment of pediatric major depressive disorder (poster) / C. L. Donnelly, A. Winoker, C. J. Wohlberg // Presented at American College of Neuropsychopharmacology (ACNP) Annual Meeting. - Waikoloa, Hawaii, 2001. - Dec.

256. Drummond, M. Economic evaluation of pharmanticals : Science or marketing? / M. Drummond // Pharmac. Economics. - 1992. - № 1. - P. 8—13.

257. Dugas, M. Etats depressifs chez les enfants / M. Dugas // Vie med. Enquete. - 1966. - V. 47, № 8. - P. 1013—1020.

258. Dwyrer, I. T. A family history study of twenty probands with childhood manic- depressive illness / I. T. Dwyrer, G. R. Delong // J. Am. Acad. Child. Psychiatry. - 1987. - V. 26, № 2. - P. 176-180.

259. Edeltan, G. The Remembered Present : A Biological Theory of Consciousness / G. Edeltan. - N. Y. : Basic Bookc, 1989. - P. 44.

260. Eggers, Ch. Childhood depression under developmental psychological aspects / Eggers Ch. // Acta paedopsychiat. - 1980/81. V. 46. P. 263-273.

261. Eley, T. C. Parental vulnerability, family environment and their interactions as predictors of depressive symptoms in adolescents / T. C. Eley, H. Liang, R. Plomin, P. Sham, A. Sterne, R. Williamson, S. Purcell // J. of the American Academy of Child and Adolescent Psychiatry. - 2004. - V. 43. - P. 298—306.

262. Ellis, A. Reason and emotion in psychotherapy / A. Ellis. - N. Y. : Lyle Stuart, 1962.

263. Ellis, N. R. Research perspectives in mental retardation / N. R. Ellis, A. R Cavalier // Ment. Retardation : The developmental difference controversy. - Hillsdale, 1982. - P. 121—152.

264. Emmingnaus, G. The mental disorders of childhood / G. Emmingnaus. - Tubingen, 1887 - P. 22-272.

265. Emslie G. J. Paroxetine treatment in children and adolescents with major depressive disorder : a randomized, multicenter, double-blind, placebo-controlled trial / G. J. Emslie // Nord. J. Psychiatry. - 2006. - V. 60, № 3. - P. 220-226.

266. Farlet, M. Traite de'hypochondrie et du suicide / M. Farlet. - Paris, 1822. - P. 66—67.

267. Fawcett, J. The long-term management of bipolar disorders with lithium, carbamasepine, and antidepressants / J. Fawcett, H. Kravitz // J. Clin. Psychiatry. - 1985. - V. 46, № 2. - P. 58-64.

268. Fereira, A. J. The Pregnant Womens Emotional Attitude / A. J. Fereira // Am. J. of Orthopsychiatry. - 1980. - V. 30. - P. 553—556.

269. Fineberg, N. Does childhood and adult obsessive compulsive disorder

(OCD) respond the same way to treatment with serotonin reuptake inhibitors (SRIs) / N. Fineberg, I. Heyman, R. Jenkins et al. // The Journal of the European College of Neuropsychopharmacology. - 2004. - V. 14. - Suppl. 3. - P. 191.

270. Fleming, J. T. Prevalence of childhood and adolescent depression in the community / J. T. Fleming, D. R. Offord, M. H. Boyle // Br. J. Psychiat. - 1989. - V. 155. - P. 644—654.

271. Fleming, J. The outcome of adolescent depression in the Ontario Child Health Study follow-up / J. Fleming, M. Boyle, D. Offord // J. of the American Academy of Child and Adolescent Psychiatry. - 1993. - V. 32. - P. 28—33.

272. Foa, E. Differentiation depression and anxiety : is it possible? is it useful? / E. Foa, U. Foa // Psychopharmac. Bull. - 1982. - V. 18, № 4. - P. 62-68.

273. Fowlie, M. Quality of life - a review of the literature. Family practice / M. Fowlie, I. Berheby // Social indicators research. - 1987. - V. 4, № 3. - P. 226-234.

274. Frame, C. Behavioral treatment of depression in a prepubertal child / C. Frame et al. // J. Behav. Therapy and Exper. Psychiat. - 1982. - V. 13. - P. 239—243.

275. Frangois, B. Treatment of only detected patients versus treatment of the whole population at risk of disease : a method of cost analysis applicable at the district level of health care / B. Frangois, B. Bujardin, G. Kegels // Bulletin BO3. - 1993. - T. 71, № 5. - C. 94—101.

276. Fredman, R. C. Family history of illness in seriously suicidal adolescents : A life-cycle approach / R. C. Fredman // Am. J. Of Ontopsychiatry. - 1984. - V. 54, № 3. - P. 390-397.

277. Fries, M. E. Longitudinal Study : Prenatal Period to Parenthood / M. E. Fries // J. of American Psychoanalytic Association. - 1987. - V. 25. - P. 115—140.

278. Frommer, B. Indications for Antidepressant Treatment with Special Reference to Depressed Preschool Children / B. Frommer // Depressive States in Childhood and Adolescence. - Stockholm, 1972. - P. 449—454.

279. Garfaer, J. Recurrent depression in adolescents : a follow-up study / J. Garfaer, M. Kriss, M. Koch et al. // J. of American Academy of Child and Adolescent Psychiatry. - 1988. - V. 27. - P. 49—54.

280. Garrison, C. Z. Major Depressive Disorder and Dysthymia in Young Adolescents / C. Z. Garrison, C. L. Addy, K. L. Jackson et al. // Am. J. Epidemiol. - 1992. - V. 135. - P. 792—802.

281. Gibson, R. W. Planning a total treatment program for the hospitalized depressed patient / R. W. Gibson // Depression : biology, psychodynamics, and treatment / ed. I. O. Cjll, A. F. Shatzberg, S. H. Frazier. - New York : Plenum Press, 1978.

282. Girard, J. La cephalee d'attention comme symptome de depression chez

l'enfant / J. Girard // Depressive States in Childhood and Adolescence. - Stockholm, 1972. - P. 187—200.

283. Glaser, K. Masked Depression in Children and Adolescents / K. Glaser // Am. J. Psychother. - 1967. - V. 21, № 7. - P. 565-574.

284. Glaser, K. Psychopathologic Patterns in Depressed Adolescents / K. Glaser // Am. J. Psychother. - 1981. - V. 35, № 3. - P. 368-382.

285. Goldstein, R. B. Psychiatricdisorders in relatives of probands with panic disorders and? or major depression / R. B. Goldstein, M. M. Weissman, P. B. Adams, E. Horwath, J. D. Lish, D. Charney, S. W. Woods, C. Sobin, P. J. Wickramaratne // Arch. Gen. Psychiatry. - 1994. - V. 51. - P. 383—394.

286. Goldstein, T. R. History of suicide attempts in pediatric bipolar disorder : factors associated with increased risk / T. R. Goldstein, B. Birmaher, D. Axelson et. al. // J. Bipolar Disord. - 2005. - Dec. - V. 7, № 6. - P. 525-535.

287. Gollnitz, G. Zusaimnentang von fruhkindlicher Encephalopatie und depressiven Zustanden / G. Gollnitz // Depressive States in Childhood and Adolescende. - Stockholm, 1972. p. 227-232.

288. Goodyer, I. Short-term outcome of major depression : II. Life events, family dysfunction, and friendship difficulties as predictors of persistent depression / I. Goodyer, J. Herbert, A. Tamplin, S. M. Secher, J. Pearson // J. Am. Child. Adolesc. Psychiatry. - 1997. - V. 36. - P. 474.

289. Gorboz, R. Are there mental diseases in childhood / R. Gorboz // Schwies. Med. weekly - 1958. v. 88. p. 703-712.

290. Gothelf, D. Pilot study : fluvoxamine treatment for depression and anxiety disorders in children and adolescents with cancer / D. Gothelf et al. // J. Am. Acad. Child. Adolesc. Psychiatry. - 2005. - Dec. - V. 44, № 12. - P. 1258—1262.

291. Gotlib, I. H. Treatment of depression : An interpersonal system approach / I. H. Gotlib, C. A. Cobly. - N. Y. : Pergamon, 1987.

292. Griesinger, W. Mental illness / W. Griesinger / translated from German. - SPb., 1886.

293. Hack, M. Effect of very low birth and subnormal head size on cognitive abilities at school age / M. Hack et al. // N. Engl. J. Ved. - 1991. - Jul. - V. 325, № 4. - P. 231-237.

294. Hales, D. P. Factorial validity and invariance of the center for epidemiologic studies depression (CES-D) scale in a sample of black and white adolescent girls / D. P. Hales, R. K. Dishman, R. W. Motl, C. L. Addy, K. A. Pfeiffer, R. R. Pate // Ethnicity & Disease. - 2006. - V. 16, № 1. - P. 1-8.

295. Harrington, M. Depression in girls during latency / M. Harrington, J. Hassan // Brit. J. med. Psychol. - 1958. - V. 31, № 1. - P. 43—50.

296. Harrington, R. The assessment of lifetime psychopathology : a comparison of two interviewing styles / R. Harrington, J. Hill, M. Rutter et al. //

Psychological Medicine. - 1988. - V. 18. - P. 487—493.

297. Hazerll, P. Tricyclic antidepressants for depressive disorders in children and adolescents / P. Hazerll, D. O'Connell, D. Heathcote, D. Henry // The Cochrane Library, Issue 2. - Oxford : Update Software, 2001.

298. Hazzon, D. W. Plazmacoeconomiks : Quality us of quality medicines and its impact on the Middle East / D. W. Hazzon, F. R. Plazm // International Pharmacy Journal. - 1995. - V. 9, № 4. - P. 161-162.

299. Heisel, J. St. The significance of life events as contributing factors in the diseases of children / J. St. Heisel, S. Ream, R. Raitz et al. // J. Pediatr. - 1973. - V. 83. - P. 119—123.

300. Hershberg, S. G. Anexiety and depressive disorders in psychiatrically disturbed children / S. G. Hershberg, G. A. Carlson, D. P. Cantwell, M. Strober // J. Clin. Psychiat. - 1982. - V. 138, № 9. - P. 358—361.

301. Hombyrger, A. Vorlesunqen uber die Psychopatoloqic des Kindesalters / A. Hombyrger. - Berlin, 1926.

302. Hunt, J. V. Very low birth weight infants at 8 and 11 years of age : role of neonatal illness and family status / J. V. Hunt et al. // Pediatrics. - 1988. - Oct. - V. 8214. - P. 596—603.

303. Hutton, S. Economic evaluation of leatth cuse : A half - way technology / S. Hutton // Health Economics. - 1994. - № 3. - P. 1—4.

304. Isacsson, G. Do SSRIs induce suicide? A controlled study of Swedish suicides 1992-2000 / G. Isacsson, P. Holmgren, J. Ahlner // The J. of the European College of Neuropsychopharmacology. - 2004. - V. 14. - Suppl. 3. - P. 145.

305. Ivarsson, T. The Children's Depression Inventory (CDI) as measure of depression in Swedish adolescents. A normative study / T. Ivarsson // BMC Psychiatry. - 2006. - May. - V. 246, № 1. - P. 24.

306. Johanneson, M. On the discounting of gained life - years in cost effectiveness analysis / M. Johanneson // Int. J. of technology assessment in health care. - 1992. - V.8, № 2. - P. 359-364.

307. Kaizar, E. E. Do antidepressants cause suicidality in children? / E. E. Kaizar // A Bayesian meta-analysis. - 2006. - Jul.-Aug. - V. 30, № 6. - P. 561-577.

308. Kandel, D. B. Epidemiology of depressive mood in adolescents an empirical study / D. B. Kandel, M. Davies // Arch. Gen. Psychiat. - 1982. - V. 39. - P. 1205—1212.

309. Kandel, D. Adult sequelae of adolescent depressive symptoms / D. Kandel, M. Davies // J. Arch. Gen. Psychiatry. - 1986. - V. 43. - P. 255—262.

310. Kashani, J. H. Depression in Children and Adolescents with Cardiovascular Symptomatology : The Significance of Chest Pain / J. H. Kashani, Z. Zababidi, R. S. Jones // J. Am. Acad. Child. Psychiat. - 1982. - V. 21, № 1. - P. 187-189.

311. Kashani, J. H. Incidence of depression in children / J. H. Kashani, J. P. Simonds // Am. J. Psychiat. - 1979. - V. 136. - P. 1203—1205.

312. Kashani, J. H. Depression in hospitalized pediatric patients / J. H. Kashani, G. J. Barber, F. D. Bolander // J. Am. Acad. Child. Psychiat. - 1981. - V. 20, № 1. - P. 123-134.

313. Kashani, J. H. Depression in Children and Adolescence with Cardiovascular Symptomatology : The Significance of Chest Pain / J. H. Kashani, G. J. Barber, F. D. Bolander // J. Am. Acad. Child. Psychiat. - 1982. - V. 21, № 1. - P. 187- 189.

314. Kashani, J. H. Depression, depressive symptoms, and depressed mood among a community sample of adolescents / J. H. Kashani, G. A. Carson, N. C. Beck et al. // Am. J. of Psychiatry. - 1987. - V. 144. - P. 931—934.

315. Katon, W. Depression and somatization : A review / W. Katon, A. Kleinman, G. Rosen // Am. J. Med. - 1982. - V. 72, № 2. - P. 241—247.

316. Katz, J. Depression in the young child / J. Katz // Modern Perspectives in the Psychiatry of infancy / ed. J. G. Howells. - New York, 1979. - P. 435—449.

317. Keller, M. Course of major depression in non-referred adolescent : a retrospective stady / M. Keller, W. Beardslee et al. // J. Affect. Disord. - 1988. - V. 15. - P. 235—243.

318. Kellner, R. The relationship of depressive neurosis to anxiety and somatic symptoms / R. Kellner, G. Simpson, W. Winslow // Psychosomatics. - 1972. - V. 13. - P. 358—367.

319. Kennneth, S. Major Depression and Generalized Anxiety Disorder (Same Genes, (Partly) Different Environments?) / S. Kennneth, M. D. Kendler et al. // Arch. Gen. Psychiatry. - 1992. - V. 49. - P. 716—722.

320. Kestenbaum, C. J. Children at risk for manic-depressive illness : possible predictors / C. J. Kestenbaum // Am. J. Psychiat. - 1979. - V. 136, № 9. - P. 1206—1208.

321. Kielholz, P. Uber 24. drug addiction in adolescents / P. Kielholz, D. Ladewig // Dtsch. med. wschr. - 1970. - V. 95. - P. 101.

322. Kielholz, P. Depressive illness / P. Kielholz. - Baltimore, 1972. - 302 p.

323. Kielholz, H. A. Le noyau depressif / Kielholz H. A. // Rev. Med. - 1980. - V. 21, № 2. - P. 77—82.

324. Klein, M. Emotional life and Ego development of the infant, with special reference to the depressive position / Klein M. // Controlv. Ser. London Psychoanal Soc. - 1944. - P. 144—150.

325. Klein, M. The paychogenesis of manic-depressive states / M. Klein // Conttributions to Psycho-Analysis. - London : Hogarth, 1934. -282 p.

326. Kohler, C. Depressive States in Childhood and Adolescence / C. Kohler, F. Bernard. - Stockholm, 1972. - P. 173—184.

327. Kohler, C. Les etats depressifs chez 1 enfant / C. Kohler, F. Bernard. - Brussels, 1970.

328. Kolvin, I. Classification and diagnosis of depression in school phobia / I.

Kolvin, T. P. Berney, S. R. Bhate // Brit. J. Psychiat. - 1984. - V. 145. - P. 347— 357.

329. Kovacs, M. An empirical approach toward a definition of childhood depression / M. Kovacs, A. T. Beck // Depression in childhood : Diagnosis, treatment and conceptual models / eds. J. G. Schulterbrandt, A. Raskin. - N. Y. : Raven Press, 1977. - P. 1—25.

330. Kovacs, M. Internalizing Disorders in Childhood / M. Kovacs, B. Devlin // J. Child. Psychol. Psychiatr. - 1998. - V. 39, № 1. - P. 47—63.

331. Kovacs, M. The trend toward a continuous change in the age of onset of MDD in a clinical pediatric sample / M. Kovacs, C. Gatsonis // J. Psychiatr Res. - 1994. - V. 28. - P. 319—329.

332. Kovacs, M.. Depressive disorders in childhood : A longitudinal prospective study / M. Kovacs, T. Fainberg et al. // Arch. Gen. Psychiatry. - 1984. - V. 41. - P. 229—237, 463—469.

333. Kraepelin, E. Psychiatric / E. Kraepelin. - Leipzig, 1913. - Bd. 3, t. 2; Bd. 4, t. 3.

334. Kuhn, R. Uber Kindliche Depressionen und ihre Behandlung / R. Kuhn // Schweiz. Med. wschr. - 1963. - Vol. 93, № 2. - pp. 86-90.

335. Kuhn, V. Depressive States in Childhood and Adolescences / V. Kuhn, R. Kuhn // Union of European Paedopsychiatrists, IV Congress. - Stockholm, 1972. - P. 455—459.

336. Kuhn, R. The treatment of masked depression / R. Kuhn // Masked Depress., Discuss. - Bern, 1973. - P. 188—194.

337. Langmeier, J. Mental deprivation in childhood / J. Langmeier, Z. Matejcek. - Prague, 1984.

338. Larsson, B. Prevalence and short-term stability of depressive symptoms in schoolchildren / B. Larsson, L. Melin // Acta. Psychiatrica Scandinavica. - 1992. - V. 85, № 1. - P. 17-22.

339. Lebovici, S. Contribution psychoanalytic to the knowledge of depression in children and adolescents / S. Lebovici // Depressive States in Childhood and Adolescence. - Stockholm, 1972. - P. 45—52.

340. Lehman H. The clinician view of anxiety and depression / H. Lehman // J. Clinic. Psychiat. - 1983. - V. 44, № 8. - P. 3—7.

341. Lesse, S. Depression Masked by Acting-out Behaviour Paterns / S. Lesse // Am. J. Psychother. - 1974. - V. 25, № 3. - P. 352-361.

342. Lesse, S. Masked depression - the ubiquitous but unapprenated-syndrome / S. Lesse // Psyfch. J. Univ. Ottawa. - 1980. - V. 5, № 4. - P. 268-273.

343. Levinshon, P. Major depression in community adolescent : age an onset, episode duration, and time to recurrense / P. Levinshon, G. Clark et. al. // J. Am Acad Child Adolesc Psychiatry. - 1994. - V. 33. - P. 809—818.

344. Lewinsohn, P. M. Cognitive-behavioral treatment for depressed adolescents. Paper presented at the annual meeting of the American

Association of Child and Adolescent Psychiatry / P. M. Lewinsohn et al. - Washington, 1987.

345. Lewontin, R. Human individuality: heredity and environment / R. Lewontin / translated from English - M., 1993. - 208 c.

346. Lindahl, E. Motor performance risk and non-risk children at early school - age / E. Lindahl // Acta. Paediatr. Scand. - 1987. - Sep. - V. 76, № 5. - P. 809-817.

347. Ling, W. Depressive Illness in Childhood Presenting as Severe Headache / W. Ling, G. Oftedal, W. Weinberg // Am. J. Dis. Child. - 1970. - V. 120, № 2. - P. 122-124.

348. Lizshnez, B. Amitho do logical framework for assessing health indices / B. Lizshnez, G. Guyatt // J. chzon. Pis. - 1985. - V. 38, №1. - P. 27—36.

349. Loskutova, E. Development o the Optimum Drugs List For the Treatment of Psychic Disorders / E. Loskutova, V. Doroteyeva., Maximkina // Report on the 56th world Congress of Pharmacy and Pharmaceutical Sciences. - Jerusalem, 1996. - P. 101.

350. M. K. Nixon, R. Milin, J. G. Simeon et al. Child Adolesc. Psychopharmacol. 2001. - V. 11. - P. 131—42.

351. Malmquist, C. P. Depressions in childhood and adolescence / C. P. Malmquist // Engl. J. Med. - 1971. - V. 284, № 2. - P. 387-893.

352. Maloney, M. Diagnosing hysterical conversion reaction in children / M. Maloney // J. Pediatr. - 1980. - V. 97. - P. 1016—1020.

353. Maneeton, N. Tricyclic antidepressants for depressive disorders in children and adolescents : A meta-analysis of randomized-controlled trial / N. Maneeton, M. Srisurapanont // J. Med. Assoc. Trai. - 2000. - V. 83. - P. 1367—1374.

354. Marc, L. De la folie consideree dans ses, rapports avec les quesyions medico-judiciales / L. Marc Paris. - 1840. - 328 p.

355. Maris, R. M. Pathways to suicide : A survey of self-destructive behavior / R. M. Maris. - Baltimore John Hopkins University Press, 1981.

356. Marriage, K. Relationship between depression and conduct disorder in children and adolescents / K. Marriage, S. Fine, M. Mloretti, G. Haley // J. Am. Acad. Child. Psychiat. - 1986. - V. 25, № 5. - P. 687-691.

357. Marttunen, M. D. Mental disorders in adolescent suicide : DSM-III-R Axis I and II in suicide among 13-to19-year-olds in Finland / M. D. Marttunen, M. M. Henrikson et. al. // Archives of General Psychiatry. - 1991. - V. 48. - P. 834— 839.

358. Maudsley, H. Physiology and Pathology of the Soul / H. Maudsley. - St. Petersburg, 1871.

359. Mayer-Gross, W. Clinical Psychiatry / W. Mayer-Gross, E. Slater, M. Roth. - London, 1954.

360. McCauley, E. Depression in young people : initial presentation and clinical

course / E. McCauley, K. Myers, J. Mitchell et al. // J. of the American Academy of Child and Adolescent Psychiatry. - 1993. - V. 32. - P. 714—722.

361. McHolm, A. E. The relationship between childhood physical abuse and suicidality among depressed women : results from a community sample / A. E. McHolm // Am. J. Psychiatry. - 2004. - Apr. - V. 161, № 4. - P. 762-763.

362. Mcirhofer, M. Deprssive Verstimmunqen in fruhtn Kindesalter / M. Mcirhofer // Depressive states in childhood and adolescence / ed. by A. Annel // Union of European Paedop psychiatrists, IV Congress Stockholm /- 1972. - P. 159—162.

363. Medow, W. Atipische Psychsen bei Oligophrenie / W. Medow // Monatsschrift fur Psychiatrie und Heurologie. - Berlin, 1925. vol. LUIII, h. 5. pp. 289-323.

364. Meichenbaum, D. Cognitive behavior modification / D. Meichenbaum. - N. Y. Plenum, 1977.

365. Mendelson, W. B. Some Characterististic Features Accompanying Depression, Anxiety and Aggressive Behaviour in Disturbed Children under Five / W. B. Mendelson, M. A. Reid, E. A. Frommer // Depressive States in Childhood and Adolescence. - Stockholm, 1972. - P. 151—158.

366. Mick, E. Effectiveness of risperidone for the treatment of ADHD in children and adolescents with bipolar disorder European Neuropsychopharmacology / E. Mick, J. Biederman // The J. of the European College of Neuropsychopharmacology. - 2004. - V. 14. - Suppl. 3. - P. 212.

367. Miller, K. Suicidal adolescents' perceptions of their family environment / K. Miller, C. King, B. Shain, M. Naylor // Suicide and Life-Threatening Behavior. - 1992. - V. 22, № 2. - P. 227-229.

368. Moreau de Tours, J. La folie chez l'enfant / J. Moreau de Tours. - Paris, 1888.

369. Moreau de Tours, P. De la demence dans ses rapports avec l'eteat normal des facultes intellectuelles et affectives / P. Moreau de Tours. - Paris, 1888. - P. 13— 16, 28, 68, 81—87, 294—319, 392—393.

370. Moreau de Tours, P. De la folie jalousie / P. Moreau de Tours. - Paris, 1877.

371. Murray, P. A. The clinical picture of depression in school-cildren / P. A. Murray // J. Irish. Med. Assoc. - 1970. - V. 63, № 392. - P. 53—56.

372. Negri, M. De Quelques aspects de depressions infantiles / M. De Negri, G. Morett // Acta Paedopsychiat. - 1972. - V. 38, № 7—8. - P. 182—190.

373. Neustadt, R. The psychoses of the feeble-minded / R. Neustadt. - Berlin, 1928.

374. Nissen, G. Antidepressant infusions in juvenile oaks / G. Nissen // Antidepressant infusion therapy / eds P. Kielholz, C. Adams. - Stuttgart, New York : G. Thieme, 1982. pp. 50-53.

375. Nissen, G. Das depressive Syndrome im Kindes - und Jugendalter / G. Nissen // hrsg. H. Hippius, W. Janzarik, M. Muller. - Berlin, Hidelberg, New

York, 1971. - - 174 s.

376. Nissen, G. Depression in childhood and adolescence / G. Nissen // Triangle. - 1982. - V. 21, №2-3. - P. 77-83.

377. Nissen, G. Depression and suicidality in adolescence / G. Nissen // Z. Allgemeinaed. Landarzt. - 1973. vol. 49, № 10. pp. 435-440.

378. Nissen, G. Depressive and hypochondriacal disorders in childhood / G. Nissen // Prax. Kinderpsychol. - 1987. V. 6-14. P. 16.

379. Nissen, G. Larvierte Depressionen bei Kindern / G. Nissen // Acta Paedopsychiat. - 1975. - V. 41, № 6. - P. 235—241.

380. Nissen, G. Masked depression in children and adolescents / G. Nissen // Masked depression / ed. By P. Kielholz. - Bern, Stuttgart, Vienna, 1973. - P. 144—149.

381. Nissen, G. Masked depressions in children and adolescents / G. Nissen // Masked Depression / ed. P. Kielholz. - Bern, Stuttgart, Vienna : H. Huber Publishers, 1973. - P. 133—143.

382. Nissen, G. Milia factors and later schizophrenic psychosis in depressed children / G. Nissen // Arch. Psychiat. Nervenkr. - 1971. v. 214, № 4th - p. 319-323.

383. Nissen, G. Psychische storungen mit vorviegend psychische Symptomatik / G. Nissen // Textbook of special child and adolescent psychiatry / edited by U. A. von Harbauer. - Berlin, 1971.

384. Nissen, G. Special problems in the therapy of depressed children and adolescents / G. Nissen // Avoidable errors in diagnosis and therapy of depression / hrg. P. Kielholz, C. Adams. - Koln : Deusch. Arzte, 1984. pp. 121-125.

385. Nissen, G. Symtomatik und Prognose depressiver veretimmungzustande in Kindesund Jugendalter / G. Nissen // Depressive states in childhood and adolescence : Union of European Paedopsychiatrists, IV Congress / ed. by A. Annel. - Stockholm. 1972. - P. 501—509.

386. Nissen, G. T. Masked depressions in children and adolescents / G. T. Nissen // Masked Depression / ed. P. Kielholz. - Bern, Stuttgart, Vienna : H. Huber Publishers, 1973. - P. 133—143.

387. Nissen, G. On the classification of dopressions in childhood / G. Nissen // Acta. paedopsychiat. - 1980/81. - Vol. 46, № 5-6. - pp. 275-284.

388. Nissen, G. Is depression masked in children? / G. Nissen // J. Acta paedopsychiatr. - Baseel, 1975. - V. 41, № 6. - P. 235—242.

389. Panthiratphom, Ch. Pernatel Infant Stimulation Program / Ch. Panthiratphom // Prenatal Recertion / ed. D. Blum. - N. Y., 1994. - P. 187—220.

390. Petrou, S. The reliability of cost-utility estimates in cost-QALY league tables / S. Petrou, M. Malek, P. G. Pavey // Pharmaco Economics. - 1993. - № 3. - P. 345—353.

391. Petti, T. A. Evaluation and multimodality treatment of a depressed prepubertal girl / T. A. Petti et al. // J. Acad. Child Psychiat. - 1980. - V 19. - P. 690—702.

392. Pfeffer, C. R. Suicidal children grow up : relations between family psychopathology and adolescents' lifetime suicidal Behavior / C. R. Pfeffer, L. Normadin, T. Kakuma // J. of nervous and Mental Disease. - 1998. - V. 186. - P. 269—275.

393. Philips, I. Childhood depression : interpersonal interactions and depressive phenomena / I. Philips // Am. J. Psychiat. - 1979. - V 136, № 48. - P. 511—515.

394. Pine, D. The risk for early adulthood anxiety and depressive disorders in adolescents with anxiety and depressive disorders / D. Pine, P. Cohen, D. Gurley et al. /I Archives of General Psychiatry. - 1998. - V. 55. - P. 56—64.

395. Pinel, Ph.D. Medical-philosophical treatment of alienation or mania / Ph. Pinel. - Paris, 1809.

396. Pinkerton, Ph. Depression and Denial in Childhood Asthma : Equipotent Fatal Hazards / Ph. Pinkerton // Depressive States in Childhood and Adolescence. - Stockholm, 1972. - P. 187—192.

397. Poznanski, S. A depression rating scale for children / S. Poznanski, S. C. Cook, B. J. Carroll // Pediatrics. - 1979. - V. 64, № 4. - P. 442-450.

398. Poznanski, E. Childhood Depression. Longitudinale Perspective / E. Poznanski, V. Krahenbuhe, J. P. Zrubl // J. Child. Psychiat. - 1976. - V. 15, № 3. - P. 491—501.

399. Puig-Antich, J. A controlled family history study of prepubertal major depressive disoders / J. Puig-Antich, D. Goetz et al. // Arch. Gen. Psychiatry. - 1989. - V. 46. - P. 406—418.

400. Puig-Antich, J. The diagnosis and treatment of major depressive disorder in childhood / J. Puig-Antich, B. Weston // Ann. Rev. Med. - 1983. - № 34. - P. 231—245.

401. Puig-Antich, J. The use of RDC criteria for major depressive disorder in children and adolescents / J. Puig-Antich // J. Am. Acad. Child. Psychiat. - 1982. - V. 21, № 3. - P. 291-293.

402. Puzynska, E. The course of affective diseases of the endogenous type in children and adolescents / E. Puzynska, M. Mazurczak // Psychiat. Pol. - 1978. - V. 12, № 3. - P. 341—347.

403. Quay, H. C. Dimensions of personality in delinquent boys as inferred from the factor analysis of case history data / H. C. Quay // Child. Developm. - 1964. - V. 35. - P. 473—484.

404. Quellete-Kuntz, H. A pilot study in the use of the quality of life interview schedule / H. Quellete-Kuntz // Social indicators research. - 1990. - V. 23, № 3. - P. 238-298.

405. Rao, U. Depression as a risk factor for suicide : preliminary report of

longitudinal study / U. Rao, B. Weissman, J. A. Martin, R. W. Hammond // J. Am. Acad. Child. Adolesc. Psychiatry. - 1993. - V. 31. - P. 21—28.

406. Rao, U. Unipolar depression in adolescents : clinical outcome in adulthood / U. Rao, N. Ryan, B. Birmaher et al. // J. of the American Academy of Child and Adolescent Psychiatry. - 1995. - V. 34. - P. 466—578.

407. Rapee, R. M. The potential role of childrearing practices in the development of anxiety and depression / R. M. Rapee // Clin. Psychol. Rev. - 1997. - V. 17. - P. 47—67.

408. Remschmidt, H. On the course of illness and perzonlichkeitsstructur of children and adolescents with endogenpfasichen psychoses and reactiven Depressionen / H. Remschmidt, B. Bretchel, F. Mewe // Acta Paedopsychiatr. - 1973. - Vol. 40. - P. 2-13.

409. Remschmidt, H. On the course of illness and the personality structure of children and adolescents with engagenic-phase psychoses and reactive depression / H. Remschmidt, B. Brechtel, F. Mewe // Acta Paedopsychiat. - 1973. V. 40, № 1ST - P. 2-17.

410. Renshaw, D. C. Suicide and depression in children / D. C. Renshaw // J. School Hlth. - 1974. - V. 44, № 3. - P. 487-489.

411. Reyes-Harde, M. Risperidone in children with disruptive behavior disorders : A 2-year open-label trial European Neuropsychopharmacology / M. Reyes-Harde, J. Croonenberghs, M. Eerdekens // J. European College of europsychopharmacology. - 2004. - V. 14. - Suppl. 3. - P. 274.

412. Reynolds, W. M. A comparison of cognitive-behavioral therapy and relaxation training for the treatment of depression in adolescents / W. M. Reynolds, K. I. Coats // J. Consult. Clin. Psychol. - 1986. - V. 54. - P. 653—660.

413. Rich, C. L. San Diego suicide study : The adolescents / C. L. Rich, M. Sherman, R. C. Fowler, Adolescence. - 1990. - V. 25. - P. 855—865.

414. Rie, H. E. Depression in childhood : a survey of some persinent contributions / H. E. Rie // J. Am. Acad. Child. Adolesc. Psychiatry. - 1966. - V. 5. - P. 653— 685.

415. Rinsley, D. B. Intensive psychiatric hospital treatment of adolescents. An object-relations view / D. B. Rinsley // Psychiat. Quart. - 1965. - V. 39, № 3. - P. 405-429.

416. Rjchlin, G. The lost complex : the contribution to the etiology of depression / G. Rjchlin // J. Am. Psychoanal. Assoc. - 1969. - V. 7. - P. 293—316.

417. Robbins, D. R. The use of Research Diagnostic Criteria (RDC) for depression in adolescent psychiatric inpatients / D. R. Robbins, N. E. Alees, S. C. Cook, et al. // J. Am. Acad. Child. Psychiat. - 1988. - V. 21. - P. 251—255.

418. Runeson, B. Mental disorder in youth suicide : DSM-III-R Axes I and II / B. Runeson // Fcta Psych. Scandinavica. - 1989. - V. 79. - P. 490—497.

419. Runeson, B. Yonth suicides unknown to psychiatric care provides / B. Runeson // Suicide and Life-Threatening Behavior. - 1992. - V. 22, № 4. - P. 494-503.

420. Rutter, M. L. Adolescent turmoil : fact of fiction / M. L. Rutter, P. Graham, O. F. D. Chadwick, W. Yule // J. Child. Psychol. Psychiat. - 1976. - V. 17, № 1. - P. 35-56.

421. Rutter, M. L. Relationships between child and adult psychiatric disorders / M. L. Rutter // Act. Psychiat. - 1972. - V. 2, № 3. - P. 3-21 .

422. Rutter, M. L. Stress, coping and development : some issues and some questions / M. L. Rutter // J. of Child Psychology and Psychiatry. - 1981. - V. 22. - P. 223—256.

423. Salle, F. R. Pulse intravenous clomipramine for depressed adolescents : double-bild, controlled train / F. R. Salle, N. S. Vrindavanam, D. Deas-Nesmith, S. W. Carson, G. T. Sethuraman // Am. J. Psychiatry. - 1997. - V. 154. - P. 668—673.

424. Schachter, M. Study of depressions and depressive episodes in children and adolescents / M. Schachter // Acta. Paedopsychiatr. - 1972. - V. 38. - P. 131—143.

425. Schaffer, D. A critical note on the predictive validity of the hyperkinetic syndrome / D. Schaffer, L. Greenhill // J. Child. Psychol. Pcychiat. - 1979. - V. 20, № 1. - P. 61-72.

426. Schmitz, W. Decline in school performance as a primary symptom of endogenous depression / W. Schmitz // Depressive States in chidrenhood and Adolescence. - Stocrholm, 1972. h. 263-268.

427. Scott, W. C. M. A psychoanalytic concept of the origin of depression / W. C. Scott // Br. Med. J. - 1948. - V. 1, № 4550. - P. 538—540.

428. Shaffer, D. Depression, Mania and Suicidal Acts / D. Shaffer // J. Am. Acad. Child. Adolesc. Psychiatry. - 1996. - V. 44. - P. 698—708.

429. Shaffer, D. Psychiatric diagnosis in child and adolescent suicide / D. Shaffer, P. Fisher, P. Trautman et. al. // Archives of General Psychiatry. - 1996. - V. 53. - P. 339—348.

430. Shiryaev, O. Clinical-social characteristics of children and teenagers that made suicidal attempt / O. Shiryaev, A. Neretina, G. Kosheleva, I. Mahortova // J. Psychiatr. Danub. - 2006. - Sep. - V. 18. - P. 150.

431. Slap, G. Adoption as a risk factor for attempted suicide during adolescence / G. Slap G., E. Goodman, B. Huang // Pediatrics. - 2001. - V. 108, № 2. - P. 30.

432. Spiel ,W. The endogenous psychoses of childhood and adolescence / W. Spiel. - New York, Basle : Karger, 1961. 182 p.

433. Spiel, W. Melancholic in research, minik and treatment / W. Spiel / edited by W. Schulte, W. Mtndle. - Stuttgart, 1969. p. 208-210.

434. Spiel, W. Studien ber den Erscheinungsformen der Kindlichen und

juvenilen manisch-depressiven Psychosen / W. Spiel // Depressive states in childhood and adolescence. - Stockholm, 1972. p. 517-524.

435. Spitz, R. A. Anaclitic depression : an inquiry into the genesis of psychiatric conditions in early childhood / R. A. Spitz, K. M. Wolf // J. Psychoanal. Stud. Child. - 1946. - V. 51, № 2. - P. 313-342.

436. Spitz, R. A. Hospitalizm. An inquiry into the genesis of psychiatric conditions in early childhood / R. A. Spitz // J. Psychoanal. Stud. Child. - 1945. - V. 1. - P. 53.

437. Spitz, R. A. Infantile depression and general adaptation syndrome / R. A. Spitz // Crianga Port. - 1960. - V. 19. - P. 55—73.

438. Spitz, R. A. Vom S'uglingzum Kleinkind / R. A. Spitz // Natural history of mother-child relationships in the first year of life. - Stuttgart : Klett, 1967.

439. Spitz, R. A. Psychoanalytic Study of the Child / R. A. Spitz, K. M. Wolf. - N. Y., 1946. - P. 13.

440. Stadeli, H. Chronic depression in children and adolescents / H. Stadeli. - Bern, Stuttgart, Vienna : Huber, 1978. - 165 p.

441. Stark, K. D. A comparison of the relative efficacy of self-control therapy and a behavioral problem-solving therapy for depression in children / K. D. Stark, W. M. Reynolds, N. J. Kaslow // J. Child Psychol. - 1987. - V. 15. - P. 91—113.

442. Stark, K. D. Treatment of depression during childhood and adolescence : Cognitive-behavioral procedures for the individual and the family / K. D. Stark, L. W. Rouse, R. Livingston // Child and adolescent therapy : Cognitive-behavioral procedures / ed. P. C. Kendall. - 1990.

443. Stark, K. D. Childhood depression : Theory and family - school intervention / K. D. Stark, C. S. Brookman // Handbook of family - school intervention : A system perspective / eds. M. J. Fine, C. Carlson. - Boston : Allyn & Bacon, 1992. - P. 247—271.

444. Statten, T. Depressive anxieties and their differences in childhood / T. Statten // Canad. Med. Ass. J. - 1961. - V. 84, № 15. - P. 824—827.

445. Strober, M. The course of major depressive disorder in adolescents : I. Recovery and risk of manic switching in a follow-up of psychotic and - nonpsychotic subtypes / M. Strober, C. Lampert, S. Schmidt et al. // J. of the American Academy of Child and Adolescent Psychiatry. - 1993. - V. 32. - P. 34—42.

446. Stutte, H. Epochal changes in the diagnosis and course of endogenous depressive psychoses in childhood / H. Stutte // Depressive states in childhood and adolescend. - Stockholm, 1972. p. 29-34.

447. Tincolini, V. G. Depression et ambivalence / V. G. Tincolini, P. Toschi // Depressive States in Childhood and Adolescence. - Stockholm, 1972. - P. 412— 419.

448. Tolstrup, K. Psychosomatic aspects of fatness in childhood / K. Tolstrup //

Psyche. - 1963. V. 16, № 3. P. 592.

449. Toolan, F. Neurosis and psychosis in adolescent / F. Toolan // Triangle. - 1971. - V. 29. - P. 89—96.

450. Toolan, J. M. Depressions in children and adolescent / J. M. Toolan // Am. J. Orthopsychiat. - 1962. - V. 32, № 3. - P. 404-415.

451. Toolan, J. M. Suicide in children and adolescents / J. M. Toolan // Am. J. Psychiat. - 1975. - V. 29, №3. - P. 339—344.

452. Torgersen, S. Comorbidity of major depression and anxiety disorders in twin pairs / S. Torgersen // Am. J. Psychiatry. - 1990. - V. 147. - P. 1199—1202.

453. Van Praag, H. M. Depression, anxiety disorders, aggression : attempts to untangle the Gordian knot / H. M. Van Praag // Mediography.- 1998. - T. 20, № 2. - C. 27—35.

454. Varsamis, J. Manic-depressive disease in childhood. A case report / J. Varsamis, S. M. McDonald // Cand. Psychiat. Ass. J. - 1972. - V. 17, № 4. - P. 279-281.

455. Von Kroff, M. Anxiety and depression in primary care clinic : comparison of DIS, GHQ and practitioner assessments / M. Von Kroff, S. Shapiro, J. D. Burke et al. // Arch. Gen. Psychiatry, 1987. - 44. - P. 152—156.

456. Vernu, T. R. Predinite Psychology: An Introduction / T. R. Vernu. - N. Y. Human Science Press, 1987. - P. 25.

457. Wagner, K. D. Sertraline Pediatric Depression Study Group. Efficacy of sertraline in the treatment of children and adolescents with major depressive disorder : two randomized controlled trials / K. D. Wagner, P. Ambrosini, M. Rynn et al. // J. Am. Med. As. - 2003. - V. 290. - P. 1033—1041.

458. Wagner, K. D. Yang Efficacy of sertraline in an anxious subgroup of youths with major depression / K. D. Wagner, J. Ambrosini, R. Gillespie // The Journal of the European College of Neuropsychopharmacology. - 2004. - V. 4. - Suppl. 3. - P. 186.

459. Waller, D. A. Differentiating Primary Affective Disease, Organic, Affective Syndromes, and Situational Depression on a Pediatric Service / D. A. Waller, J. A. Rush // J. Am. Acad. Child. Psychiat. - 1983. - V 22, № 1. - P. 52-58.

460. Ward, A. J. Prenatal stress and childhood psyhopatology / A. J. Ward // Child Psychiatry and Human Development. - 1991. - V. 22. - P. 97—110.

461. Wasserman, G. A. Suicide risk at juvenile justice intake / G. A. Wasserman // J. Clin. Psychopharmacol. - 2006. - Jun. - V. 26, № 3. - P. 311—315.

462. Weber, A. Cattle psychiatry / A. Weber // General and special psychiatry / edited by M. Reichardt. - Basel : V. Kargtr, 1955. - pp. 193-254.

463. Weinberg, W. A. Depression and delinquency in adolescence / W. A. Weinberg, M. van den Dungen // Depressive Shates in Childhood and Adolescence. - Stockholm, 1972. - P. 296—301.

464. Weiberg, W. A. Depression in children referred to an educational diagnostic center : diagnosis and treatment. Preliminary report / W. A. Weiberg, J. Rutman, L. Suillivan et al. // J. Pediat. - 1973. - V. 83, № 6. - P. 1065-1072.

465. Weiner, J. B. Depression in adolescence / J. B. Weiner // Psychological disturbances in adolescence. - New York : Wiler, 1970. - P. 99—117.

466. Weissman, M. Children of Depressed Parents at Higher-Risk for Mental Disorders / M. Weissman, D. Pilowsky et al. // The Am. J. of Psychiatry. - 2006. - V. 163. - P. 1001—1007.

467. Weissman, M. Depressed adolescents grown up / M. Weissman, S. Wolk, R. Goldstein et al. // J. of the Am. Med. Association. - I999. - V. 281. - P. 1707—1713.

468. Weller, E. B. Depression in children and adolescents : does gender make a difference? / E. B. Weller, A. Kloos, J. Kang., R. A. Weller // Current Psychiatry Reports. - 2006. - Apr. - V. 8, № 2. - P. 108-14.

469. Weller, R. A. Depression in recently bereaved prepubertal children / R. A. Weller, E. B. Weller, M. A. Fristad, J. M. Bowes // Am. J. Psychiatry. - 1991. - V. 148. - P. 1536—1540.

470. Wieck, Ch. Schizophrenie im Kindesalter / Ch. Wieck. - Leipzig, 1965.

471. Wiesse, J. Zur endogen-phasischen Psychose an der Schwell zur Adoleszenz / J. Wiesse, P. Mattijat // Acta Paedopsychiatrica. - 1982. - Bd. 47, № 6. - S. 341—349.

472. Witkowska-Roszka, J. Depressive syndromes in children aged 7 to 14 years / J. Witkowska-Roszka // Psychiat. Pol. - 1980. - V. 14, № 3. - P. 223—227.

473. Ziehen, J. T. Die Geisteskrankheiten des Kinfesalters / J. T. Ziehen. - Berlin, 1917.

474. Zoccolillo, M. The outcome of childhood conduct disorder : implications for defining adult personality disorder and conduct disorder / M. Zoccolillo, A. Pickles, D. Quinton et al. // Psychological Medicine. - 1992. - V. 22. - P. 971— 986.

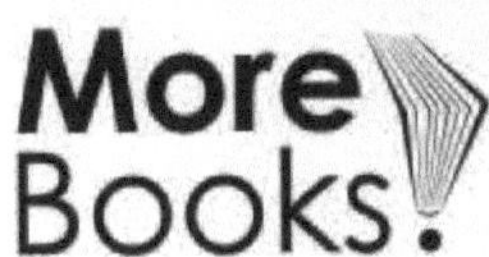

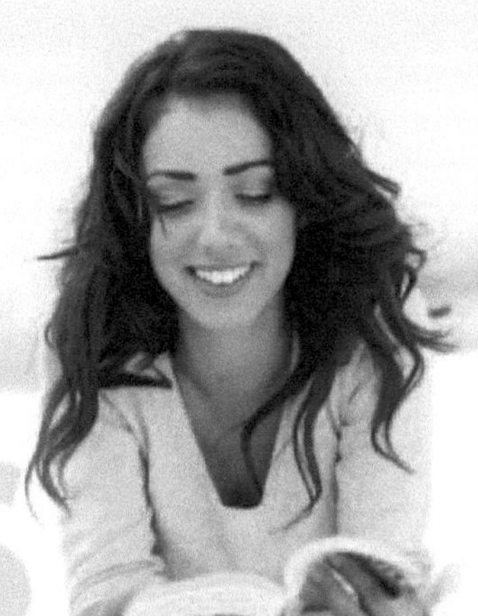

Buy your books fast and straightforward online - at one of world's fastest growing online book stores! Environmentally sound due to Print-on-Demand technologies.

Buy your books online at
www.morebooks.shop

Kaufen Sie Ihre Bücher schnell und unkompliziert online – auf einer der am schnellsten wachsenden Buchhandelsplattformen weltweit! Dank Print-On-Demand umwelt- und ressourcenschonend produzi ert.

Bücher schneller online kaufen
www.morebooks.shop

KS OmniScriptum Publishing
Brivibas gatve 197
LV-1039 Riga, Latvia
Telefax +371 686 204 55

info@omniscriptum.com
www.omniscriptum.com

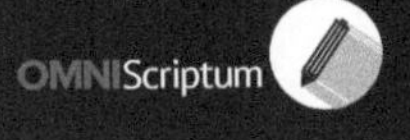

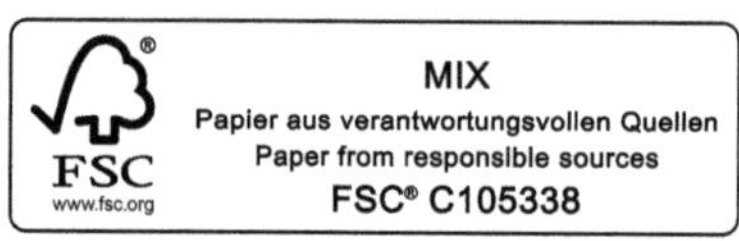

Printed by Books on Demand GmbH, Norderstedt / Germany